MANHOOD AND

Manhood and Morality explores issues of male identity among the Gisu of Uganda, within the context of the moral dilemmas faced by men who define themselves in terms of their capacity for violence.

Drawing extensively on twenty years of fieldwork experience and informed by psychological theory, Suzette Heald's discussion encompasses circumcision, ritual, witchcraft, deviance, joking, sexuality and ethnicity. In examining the power of masculinity to set the moral agenda, this ethnographic study challenges our preconceptions of manhood, inviting a wider re-evaluation of masculinity.

The book is comprised of self-contained sections, in which the narrative is contextualised within contemporary debate, providing a highly readable, user-friendly text. It makes compelling reading for students of anthropology and gender, and for all those interested in African culture.

Suzette Heald is Senior Lecturer in Anthropology at the University of Lancaster and is currently teaching at the University of Botswana.

MANHOOD AND MORALITY

Sex, violence and ritual in Gisu society

Suzette Heald

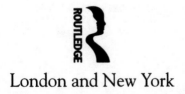

London and New York

First published 1999
by Routledge
11 New Fetter Lane, London EC4P 4EE

Simultaneously published in the USA and Canada
by Routledge
29 West 35th Street, New York, NY 10001

Typeset in Goudy by Routledge
Printed and bound in Great Britain by
Creative Print and Design (Wales), Ebbw Vale

British Library Cataloguing in Publication Data
A catalogue record for this book is available from the British Library

Library of Congress Cataloguing in Publication Data
Heald, Suzette
Manhood and morality: sex, violence and ritual in Gisu society
Includes biographical references and index
1. Gisu (African people)–Psychology. 2. Gisu (African people)–
Sexual behavior. 3. Gisu
(African people)–Rites and ceremonies.
4. Men–Uganda–Identity. 5. Sex role–Uganda–Moral and
ethical aspects. 6. Violence–Uganda. I. Title.
dt433.245.G57H45 1999
305.38'896395–dc21

ISBN 0–415–18577–7 (hbk)
ISBN 0–415–18578–5 (pbk)

For Mary Douglas

CONTENTS

CONTENTS

ACKNOWLEDGEMENTS

Grateful acknowledgement is made to the publishers for permission to reproduce the following essays, listed in order of publication:

'The making of men: the relevance of vernacular psychology to the interpretation of a Gisu ritual', *Africa* 52(1): 15–36, 1982, by permission of the International African Institute.

'The ritual use of violence: circumcision among the Gisu of Uganda', in D. Riches (ed.) *The Anthropology of Violence*, 1986: 70–85, by permission of Basil Blackwell.

'Witches and thieves: deviant motivations in Gisu society', *Man n.s.* 21(1): 65–78, 1986 and 'Joking and avoidance, hostility and incest: an essay on Gisu moral categories', *Man n.s.* 25: 377–92, 1990. Both by permission of the Royal Anthropological Institute.

'Divinatory failure: an examination of the religious and social role of Gisu diviners', *Africa* 61(1): 299–317, 1991, by permission of the International African Institute.

'Every man a hero: Oedipal themes in Gisu circumcision', in S. Heald and A. Deluz (eds) *Anthropology and Psychoanalysis*, 1994: 184–209, by permission of Routledge.

'The power of sex: some reflections on the Caldwells' "African sexuality" thesis', *Africa* 65(4): 489–505, 1995, by permission of the International African Institute.

Acknowledgement is also made to Heinemann International for permission to use quoted material from T. Wangusa, *Upon this Mountain*, 1989, in Chapter 8.

1

INTRODUCTION

This book results from a long-standing dialogue with the Gisu of Uganda, a dialogue which began in the field and proceeded through an interrogation of my fieldnotes as I have attempted to bring different forms of understanding to their life as it was lived in the late 1960s. It consists of a series of essays on the interpretation of ritual, violence, sexuality and ethnicity.

The title of the collection, *Manhood and Morality*, does not imply a consistent pairing or equation of the terms, but two interwoven perspectives found in these essays. It seems necessary to state this partly because, teaching at the moment in Botswana, my male colleagues on hearing the title of the volume collapsed into laughter and I was teased for weeks. This reaction took me aback. Why did my colleagues not see men as 'moral'? Was there something distinctive about Tswana cultural constructions of gender that prompted such mirth? True, women here, if only by their church membership and attendance, seem to have pre-empted the moral high ground and the 'youth' are seen as increasingly unaffected by the strictures of the old sexual morality and averse to taking the advice of their elders. Or was it a more general reaction? Something, perhaps, to do with the ambiguous relationship of young men in many cultures with regard to morality? If any one is going to have licence, it might be thought that it is they. But, a further factor was that these Tswana men were also academics. Was it then something in the current intellectual climate that created such an incongruous note?

With these questions on my mind, I turned again to the burgeoning new literature on masculinity. There, too, I found little in the way of an explicit moral dimension. Rather it tends to focus on the difficulties of 'being male', of living up (or more appropriately, down) to the cultural models of masculinity which are deemed to have hegemonic power (Brod, 1987; Carrigan *et al.*1987; Cornwall and Lindisfarne,

1994; Connell, 1995). Under the influence of feminism, the theme of masculinity is now seen as inseparable from power; from male dominance and from the structures of society and its serving ideologies which have ensured the legitimisation and reproduction of that power. In the realm where all discourses are deconstructed, the idea of 'moral man' dissolves from a number of angles. In so far as an upright man can be identified with the privileges exercised within the established patriarchal order, he indeed is the 'problem'. Such men cannot be seen as 'moral', for their power over women, over resources, symbolic as well as material, runs against the new ideals of gender equality and democratic egalitarianism. The *pater familias* is a very wobbly figure and can no longer stand as a repository of virtue. Indeed, the tendency in the new 'men's studies' has been to focus on the variant forms of masculinity, with gay studies at one end of the spectrum (with its drag queens and bath houses) challenging sexual stereotypes and orthodoxies, and rogue males at the other, with research into the more macho images portrayed by 'laddism' or soccer hooliganism. Ideas of masculinity, far from assuming a unitary form, are now seen as fractured into a diversity of images and lived out in a multitude of ways.

Modern trends, whatever their origin, coalesce to reflect a sociology that privileges power as an explanatory concept, rather than the old Durkheimian view of culture as a moral order. In the 1960s, when the influence of the Frankfurt school began to be felt in Anglophone scholarship, the dictum, 'the personal is political', uniting the private (and, for Marcuse, the psychic) conflict with the public one, led to a focus on political action. Over time, this has largely displaced morality as a term in sociological discourse, associated as it is with a time before the gendered nature of power became a dominant issue and thus open to direct contestation. Wherever we look, the values by which it was thought we once lived are shown to serve interests not our own. Cultural orders are displayed as a series of multi-layered perspectives; sets of resources, adopted to further the interests of particular subjects, though often beyond their knowing.

Against this trend, the anthropological call for multi-vocality, for other voices to be heard, has an ironic ring since agency – the ability of people to establish their own meanings – is constantly challenged by textual approaches which deny them the authorship of their own narratives. So, just as the 'subject' has been decentred, so too have the terms by which such subjects live. Thus 'morality', as a word, has become suspect, a possible cover for entrenched privilege. So it now seems necessary to restate that the terms in which these debates about gendered identity are played out – and continue to unravel – are essentially moral. They are about the distribution of rights and privileges; about the nature of ethical action and the arenas in which that is displayed, judged and reflected upon. They are also about the very constitution of the person. And so, unfashionably perhaps, I will keep this concept, since it covers the terrain I wish to follow better than any other. It has another advantage in that as the abstractions of academic discourse get ever more removed from the terms of life, it provides a necessary link with lived worlds and living words.

This book takes up one particular aspect of this problem, in which the power that men claim – indeed own – is problematised not only in the observer's analysis but in terms of the Gisu's own self-conceptions. Manhood and morality are indeed inimical in so far as the characteristics of men are seen to pose difficulties for moral – that is 'good' – action. The morality about which I am talking in these essays is, however, not about issues of laxity or licence. It is about the moral dilemmas faced by men, whose very definition and self-conception is in terms of a capacity for violence. What it is to be a man, a legitimate man, is the burning issue for, like any hegemonic model, it defines in turn its own deviant forms of masculinity. These can be seen to be created at both ends of the spectrum, among men seen to be without the requisite violence and in those deemed to have too much.

Each chapter engages with a different issue in anthropology but a common thread of argument runs through them. The book turns first to Gisu circumcision ritual. This ritual may be said to establish the 'problem' for, in valorising masculinity as a symbol of ethnicity, it operates to define men as 'dangerous'. Located in the nature of men, violence thus becomes a fixed point with which the Gisu grapple with the problems posed by social living. Operating in a situation which recognises little authority, either indigenous or imposed, the argument is that Gisu ethics addresses the problem of social control through the necessity for self-control. Self-assertion as the right of all men is thus coupled with restraint as the mark of the social self. This gives a particular understanding of African selfhood in the context of male egalitarianism in which the use and control of force is at the disposal of all. Most dramatically represented in the circumcision rituals (see Chapters Two–Four), it has a bearing on the reaction to crime with the criminal seen to be 'out of control' (see Chapter Five), and on the nature of divination as a *sub-rosa* technique for counteraction and vengeance (see Chapter Six). It then takes a different form in the consideration of the moral discourses embodied in kinship, sexuality and gender relationships (see Chapters Seven and Eight).

The chapters in this book all deal with a particular discourse of masculinity and its power to set the moral agenda. The general argument is that this is not necessarily in a way that is comfortable for men as the privileged gender. The attribution of violence is profoundly ambivalent. Might only sometimes equals right and, even where it does, its legitimacy and limits are open to question. As already implied, in the West, as the older codes of masculinity have come under threat, a crisis of masculinity is now more apparent than one involving women. And the attribution of men with the powers of destructive violence again provides a touchstone. In recent years, the assumption of childhood innocence has been rudely disturbed by highly publicised cases of child murderers, just as the assumption of gentle girls as opposed to unruly and truculent boys has coloured the way in which the behaviour of children is judged and punished. It is boys and not girls who fill the institutions of juvenile correction; it is men – particularly black men – and not women who fill the prisons for violent criminal offences. There is a 'crisis on our streets' shout the newspaper headlines. The police adopt the tactics of zero-tolerance, as do teachers in hard-pressed inner city schools. Both claim success, a little dent in the mounting toll of street crime. At the same time, parents, psychologists and educationalists worry about the socialisation of boys: why are they not turning out right? Parents are informed of the need for special compensatory socialisation, to make boys more like girls, that is more relational and empathetic. Teachers are urged to be less punitive in reaction to their 'naughtiness', redefining it perhaps as 'attention-deficit disorder'. And some wonder, amid all this, how, if boys are no longer to be allowed to be boys, they might at the same time preserve any pride in their masculinity?

That male violence is both lauded and feared is a commonplace in the discourses on masculinity. Often representing normative power, it is always in danger of running out of control into marginal, transgressive and destructive forms. The interest of this particular ethnographic example is the extreme way in which violent power is located in men, a source of their rights but also, I argue, a source of self-knowledge and responsibility. As such, it forms one of the basic parameters for moral discourse, both at an explicit level as recognised in the nature of moral judgements, and in the fears which colour everyday life. The Freudian adage that 'man is wolf to man' holds also the idea that man is wolf to himself. Men fear their own violence, their own violent responses and the onus throughout, therefore, is upon self-control. The good man is one who is his own master, and can master himself as well.

In this context, it is important to stress that issues of morality are not just about the power to do good and the difficulties of so doing.

That, we might say, is the arena of the moral philosophers. More tangibly, in most social situations, they focus upon the power to do harm. Of course, such danger is not necessarily seen solely in terms of physical violence. A common African patterning is of covert female malevolence opposing overt male violence, with the latter often rendered as righteous. Indeed, going back to the Tswana example with which I started, in the course of writing I came to realise that I might have badly misinterpreted the reaction. Thinking about the Gisu, I had jumped to the wrong conclusion. For it is quite possible that the morality of men is not questioned in Botswana to anything like the same extent; indeed, men who control the public sphere are seen as the upholders of public morality and responsible action. Adulthood for both genders indeed is defined as 'being responsible' but the emphasis on female responsibility carries a symbolic load largely missing from that of men. Women's very involvement with life processes, with the hidden powers of fecundity and death – in a common southern African idiom – generates a dangerous 'heat' which is opposed to the 'cool' activities of men (Comaroff, 1985). Stereotypically, women are also associated with witchcraft.

Cultural orders are built upon such asymmetries, and it goes to the heart of personhood and agency. Yet, the Gisu example alerts us also to the different ways such asymmetries are realised. There is no necessary complementarity. Among the Gisu, we could say that the human powers of men and women are portrayed on a single scale, in which men's power of anger and destructive violence dominates the moral discourse so that they carry the burden of responsibility, and women to a large extent slip through the net. Women's fertility here is not associated with polluting power and their access to witchcraft is also deemed less harmful. Also, in this moral universe, women appear to have considerably more negotiative freedom than men, since 'harmless' if not actually equating with 'blameless', at least renders it void. For these men, who have seen through the fear of death and come out with the scars that prove it, a man is rarely held to have just cause to fear a woman.

As Howell (1997) makes clear, the idea of morality in anthropology too easily slides into a more general concept of culture. If there is a distinctive anthropological approach, it perhaps lies in the linking of moralities with indigenous ideas of the person, as first argued by Read (1955). There are, indeed, good reasons for tying morality to persons, for the standards of conduct expected of different members of a society differ, as do the evaluative modes that apply to their transgressions. The idea of double standards has become the accepted vision of patriarchal orders, with its assumption of the penalisation of women who are denied the rights and liberties of men. This, of course, goes for the Gisu as well. There too, women gain access to livelihood – in this case, land – only through their relationships to men. There too, their jural rights are curtailed. But morality is never just a matter of double standards; it always involves multiple ones, with children held less responsible than adults, and so on. In this sense, all moralities are relative, within as well as without.

In turn, as has been said, it is not just a question of responsibility, for what colours this issue more than any other is the question not of agency but of danger. Thus, a second distinctive contribution can be traced to Mary Douglas. Her (1966) theory of taboo, concentrating on the defining power of danger, was at the same time a discourse on the nature of morality. Morality could be understood as being about the good, the bad and the dangerous. Yet, the dangers of the cosmos were not invariably used to support the dominant status system; they could undermine as easily as underline. Everything, she argued, needed to be read in context, and specifically in the context of action, where concepts become tactics as they are put to multifarious uses, with sometimes ironic effects.

The chapters which follow illustrate what one might call the twists and turns of the ethnographer's task, as I have attempted to bring different forms of understanding to Gisu cultural practice. In one way or another, all the chapters deal with the paradoxes of culture, with the way schemas for living create, through the very imposition of given types of meaning, intractable moral dilemmas. These are dealt with not only at what might be called the practical level of daily life, in explicit precept and the problems of moral choice, but at an existential level in the way they are depicted in the collective texts of Gisu life, in the very patterning of kinship, as well as in belief and ritual. In an attempt to get beneath the surface, to grasp the subjective dimension in culture, the chapters all move from structural to phenomenological and psychological forms of understanding.

Yet, this very ethnographic craft leaves one at the same time with many loose ends. Partly, these derive from the themes still there in one's fieldnotes, annotated now by an attenuated set of memories. Partly, they derive from changes in disciplinary perspectives, which force one back to reconsider one's interpretations, again, and yet again. But, they also result in changes to that Gisu world itself, more influenced now by the globalising forces of modernity than they were Thirty years ago. What, for example, does one make of the recent astonishing case of a man who, in a defiant act of renunciation of his

Gisu identity, invented (and legally registered) a whole new tribe? Or, the sheer resilience of the practice of Gisu circumcision? What is the nature of the tradition which continues with such strength? And, above all, what does one make of this particular gendering of ethnicity? These are the issues that I take up in the final chapter to this volume on tribal rites and tribal rights.

2

THE MAKING OF MEN

The relevance of vernacular psychology to the interpretation of a Gisu ritual

Introduction

In 1909 the Rev. J.B. Purvis wrote of the Gisu people of Eastern Uganda that they 'distinguish themselves as a race apart from others by the name Basani, i.e., men, whilst all men of uncircumcised nations are called Basinde, i.e., boys' (Purvis, 1909: 271). In modern Uganda the idea of the Gisu as a nation of circumcised men remains as strong as ever.[1] The biennial circumcision ceremonies act as both a focus for such sentiment and a dramatic display of its power. From the blowing of horns which ushers in the circumcision year to the final aggregation ceremonies during the following December the entire ritual cycle takes about a year. The actual operations are performed in August, in strict order of clan precedence, with the clan where the practice is believed to have originated cutting their boys first. The day after, the circumcisors move to the next clan territory and so on throughout Bugisu. At their height it would be no exaggeration to claim that the festivities involve the entire population of the district – some 500,000 people – from the young children carried along with the circumcision dancing parties to the elderly who are visited as relatives of the novices, approached for guidance on ritual matters, or act as spectators. At the centre are the novices, with the ordeal of circumcision acting not only to validate their own claim to status as adult men but also to demonstrate the values of the entire community.

When a ritual has this significance for a people, it is important to inquire into what values are being affirmed and why a single ritual complex is so charged. Jean La Fontaine has addressed herself to the focal character of the rituals on a number of occasions and sought the answer in the social and, specifically, the political implications the rituals have for the individual and the community.[2] To take an example, one key feature is the fact that the rituals confer immediate

8

adult status on the initiate. He 'becomes an independent member of society and a member of his lineage on equal terms with his father' (La Fontaine, 1967: 253). This jural independence is matched by his right to economic independence; circumcision entitles him to gifts of land and bridewealth from his father, the effective wealth a man needs to establish an independent household. For the son, then, she writes, the ceremony is the 'Open Sesame to independence' (ibid.: 253), and this she has emphasised creates stress in the father and son relationship. In a system where power is related to wealth, 'the careers of father and son are linked in that they depend on the use of the same resources, and in that, as a man provides for more and more of his adult sons, so his political power diminishes' (ibid.: 254). Victor Turner, in his article on Gisu circumcision, endorses this conclusion and, more sweepingly, claims that circumcision gains its emotive force as a culturally focal symbol because it 'represents an irresoluble conflict between disparate world views. On the one hand, the universalistic and egalitarian ethos of an age-set system; and, on the other, the localised particularism and gerontocratic authoritarianism of a narrowly patrilineal system' (Turner, 1969: 243). Since age-set systems have a tendency towards gerontocracy the terms of this contrast seem odd. Nevertheless, it can be agreed that there is an opposition between the ideals of essential equality of adult men and the system of authority that is implied in patrilineal transmission and hierarchic ranking in terms of age and genealogical seniority. Such conflict undoubtedly enters into the situation of circumcision and accounts for some of the specific characteristics of the ritual, both formal and informal.

Whether circumcision draws its emotive force from such a conflict is another matter. In the British structural tradition, both La Fontaine and Turner tend to treat questions of values in terms of social-structural principles. But if this makes us wiser to the social context and politico-jural correlates of circumcision, we are no nearer understanding the specific connotations of the Gisu concept of manhood. To this end I would argue that we should take more seriously the explicit aims of the ritual. We need to ask what the Gisu perceive as happening to the boys through the ordeal of circumcision, and what change is achieved that makes the denotation 'man' appropriate thereafter.

In a number of writings, Geertz has expressed his dissatisfaction with the failure of the British structural approach to give adequate consideration and autonomy to the cultural level of belief.[3] The resulting danger is that it 'takes for granted what most needs to be elucidated' (Geertz, 1966: 42). His is a call for a more serious phenomenology where culture is seen to structure the psychological field in which the individual acts. In the particular context of *rites de passage* lack of consideration of this – the missing middle term – has led to a tendency to make a too-easy jump from ethnographic observation to classification as an instance of transition ritual without grasping the specific nature of the transition as it is perceived by the people themselves. It is, in part, a question, as Rosaldo has said, of 'giving local contexts their due account' (1980: 261). And this is not simply a matter of detail, of filling out the permutations of theme, but intrinsic to the nature of the activity. As La Fontaine (1977: 422) has commented, analyses which have followed the model set out by Van Gennep have tended to restrict the evidence to give a limited and unidimensional reading. Thus, similarity of social function – the formal conveyancing of the individual from one defined social position to another – has led to an emphasis on similarity of form. Yet the imagery of boundaries, crossings, passages and transitions which has been seen to accompany the recognition of status changes is not always enlightening. Indeed, it may lead not only to a false systematisation but prove also to provide a misleading set of metaphors. In the Gisu case, the rites do not just display a static drama of form but are more importantly concerned with a dynamic changing of the personality, powers and capabilities of the individual. The focus then should be on how the rites are *transformational*, and not merely *transitional*.

That *rites de passage* pre-suppose and entail an ontological change in the capacities of individuals was a point made many years ago by Audrey Richards in her sensitive and wide-ranging account of the Bemba *chisungu*. This, as she has made clear, has a bearing on the relevance for anthropology of a dimension which takes account of the psychology of the individual.[4] In the Durkheimian tradition the efficacy attributed to ritual – its transforming effect on the consciousness of individuals – rests ultimately on psychological process. Yet if social anthropology has largely eschewed explicit concern with psychodynamic models as outside its province of explanation, there are other ways in which a concern with psychology is clearly within the cultural domain. Here I refer to those cosmological beliefs which can be seen to contain indigenous models of psychological process. Nor, where rites explicitly aim to change or transform the individual, is this unrelated to the more general problem of ritual efficacy. Especially in the case of rituals, such as Gisu circumcision, which culminate in a painful ordeal, it would seem reasonable to suppose that the ritual process contains within itself the means of aiding the individual to undergo the ordeal successfully. Whatever else they do the rituals must at least 'work' on this level. The implication here is that not only will they have a 'pragmatic' aspect, as Richards argued, but that an examination of the psychological themes embedded in the ritual will, in giving an understanding of how the transformational process is conceived, add a necessary dimension to our understanding of its specific symbolic forms.

This chapter can be read as an essay in method and usefully compared with the sociological analyses of Gisu circumcision of La Fontaine and Turner. In arguing for priority to be given to the explicit creative aims of the rites, with the individual as subject, the question arises as to whether this will not prove as informative a frame for understanding their form and symbolism as that of latent sociological functions to which anthropology is more accustomed. La Fontaine has written that 'transformation is their manifest purpose and thus cannot, logically, be used to explain them' (1977: 422).[5] This is a view which is open to question. In taking the theme of transformation this chapter argues that we might valuably use it to reflect upon the character of the specific ritual and, more generally, to ask how far the ritual process relates to such often overt psychological aims.[6]

The themes of the ritual

Imbalu is an ordeal. It is explicitly a test of the individual requiring the greatest fortitude under extreme pain. The boy must stand absolutely still while first his foreskin is cut and then subcutaneous flesh is stripped from around the *glans penis*. The degree of pain entailed is never underplayed; the most commonly used descriptive phrases being 'fierce', 'bitter' and 'terrifying'. Only those who have faced this fact and overcome their fear can undergo the ordeal successfully. Although the Gisu no longer go to war, explicit parallels are drawn between the attitude of a warrior and that of a circumcision candidate.[7] Like a warrior, the boy must conquer his fear by convincing himself that he has the strength to overcome an enemy. This is central to the drama of circumcision. An initial focus is therefore on the way in which such feelings are encouraged in the boy and how they are assessed.

Throughout the ceremony there is the greatest concern over whether the boys have enough 'strength' (*kamani*). In the first instance this is related to physical maturity and age. Gisu boys are not considered ready for *imbalu* until well past puberty, with boys throughout most of Bugisu being circumcised within the age-range 18–25.[8] Younger boys find it extremely difficult to convince their relatives that they are ready to undergo the ordeal and are thus unlikely to be given permission. This is a critical matter, for showing cowardice not only dishonours the individual and his family but, where the boy calls out for his mother or falls to the ground during the operation, carries the potential for the destruction of his entire patriline. In such cases the boy is said to have cursed his kin. Much, then, is deemed to be at stake and the relatives must satisfy themselves that the boy is capable of undergoing the ordeal with honour. In some cases young boys are forced to extreme measures in the face of resistance by their kin. In one year, in the area in which I was working, two young boys of about fifteen both cut their own foreskins, thus forcing their fathers to bring in the circumcisors to finish the operation. This was regarded as courage of a quite exceptional order, the stuff of legend.

In the first instance, then, strength is related to physical maturity. Later it is assessed in terms of how the boy dances in the build-up to the operation. It is important to note here that this strength implies for the Gisu not only physical power but what we would call strength of purpose. The Gisu do not rigidly distinguish between qualities of mind or character and those of body. The seat of the dispositions is seen to be the heart, the strongest organ of the body. Such dispositions are made known to the world through action and speech. To say of a man that 'he speaks well' is to sum up all that is desirable in a man's bearing and attitude to others, just as it conveys the fact that he has a 'good heart'.[9] Speech as indicative of disposition takes a characteristically special form during circumcision, the boy expressing his feelings and intentions in song form alone. In no ritually marked context does he speak. The circumcision songs take a distinctive form with a solo verse line alternating with a chorus taken up by the boy's followers. The songs themselves are not sacred; rather they are of a popular character and are freely invented and elaborated upon. In general, they extol the boy's determination and his readiness to face the coming ordeal. But his determination is more evidently displayed in the vigour with which he dances.

The boy is continually exhorted *samba imbalu ni kamani* ('dance *imbalu* with strength') and *amba imbalu ni kamani* ('hold on to *imbalu* with strength'). The expressions are interchangeable, just as firmness (*xuwangala*) of intent will ultimately be manifested in the firmness of his body when he actually stands for the operation. Then he is told he must breathe normally and let his stomach muscles relax; there must be no trembling, no give-away involuntary movements of his body, twitching or even blinking of his eyes which betoken fear. The commitment required of the boy is a total one, evidenced in his complete command of his body at the time of the operation.

The sources of this commitment are two-fold: in the first place it is thought of as completely volitional; in the second it depends on the build-up of *lirima* in the boy. For the moment *lirima* may be simply glossed as 'violent emotion'. To begin with the volitional component, throughout the rituals there is a constant stress by the boy himself, his kinsmen and those officiating, that the desire for *imbalu* can come from the boy alone. He himself chooses the year in which he will be circumcised and it is repeatedly said that no one is putting any pressure on him to undergo the ordeal. So the element of social pressure (always noticeable and, in cases where a boy is considered to have dallied too long, acute), is, so to speak, erased from the record with respect to any boy who has intimated his desire to be circumcised. The plain fact is that the Gisu take pride in not tolerating uncircumcised men and those considered old enough are clearly faced with the choice of going through the operation 'voluntarily', fleeing the District or facing the prospect of being circumcised by force. I witnessed a number of instances of forcible circumcision when local feeling was running high against a few boys and they were literally seized while tending their fields or along the wayside, marched to their fathers' houses and unceremoniously cut. However, that this pressure is deemed irrelevant and asserted not to exist in the ritual context should not, I think, be taken as some kind of ritual reversal of the 'truth'. Rather its significance should be sought within the texture of the meanings created and established by the ritual.

Importantly, the desire to take *imbalu* is thought of as spiritually inspired. Boys are said to be 'caught' by the *kimisambwa kw'imbalu*, the ancestral power of *imbalu*. *Imbalu* is the most significant of the Gisu ancestral powers (sing: *kumusambwa*, pl.: *kimisambwa*) it is the only one which is universal throughout Bugisu and thus associates all Gisu with a common ancestry and the powers this is believed to transmit. The powers transmitted by the *kimisambwa* are various, most of them being associated with sickness and its control, and having also a totemic aspect. Others bequeath specific powers such as that of twinning, divination, rain-making and circumcising. The sign of being caught by a *kumusambwa* is usually a characteristic affliction which is brought under control through ritual which also serves to identify the person with the powers of that *kumusambwa*. These they exercise during life and transmit to their descendants on death. All Gisu transmit *imbalu*. It is the nature of the power they give and the special mode of transmission which distinguish the *kimisambwa* both from ordinary custom (*isambo*) perpetuated by tradition and social expectation and from ritual observance (*kimisiro*) where breach results in pollution.

The ancestral power of *imbalu* is said to catch the boys with the desire to dance. Yet, as with all the powers, this is not conceived solely as an external force which possesses the boys but rather as a potentiality now made manifest. Thus, while there are elements of what we might call possession in the sense of abnormal or special states of consciousness and feeling, the desire is seen as coming directly from the heart. The act of dancing *imbalu* is thus seen as the ultimate volitional act, the boy freely making manifest the powers to which his ancestry makes him heir. The songs of the boys and the speeches made to them by the elders reiterate this theme of volition. That the boys themselves do identify with this version of events can be illustrated in the following direct extracts from a conversation between a boy who had decided on *imbalu* trying to persuade another who was clearly wavering:

> No one has asked us to do it. No one is forcing us. We ourselves have overcome our fear. Now it is my heart itself which wants it. No one is forcing me. Father has not ordered me. It comes from my heart alone. Let me explain it this way, even though I am here talking with my friends I feel like a spirit-shadow (*cisimu*) and don't know what I am doing.
>
> It is as they tell you. It comes from your heart itself. You don't sleep but think only of *imbalu* and that if it means that I will die then I must die. You cannot say, well just let me try. For it is in your heart. It is the heart itself. It is my heart which is speaking now. Every time I hear the sound of other boys' bells I want to run and see them and my stomach trembles like that of a circumciser.[10]

The boy stresses the aspect of personal decision over and over again. Indeed the speaker, who had himself passed over several circumcision years, implies a degree of surprise at finding himself now ready for the ordeal, and that this readiness is of the kind he has been told it should be. In both extracts he also voices the strangeness of his feelings and his dissociation from his ordinary self. He feels like a disembodied spirit, *cisimu*, identified with the penumbra around the shadow, only intangibly attached to the person. Or he likens his reactions to those of the circumcisers who are caught by the *kumusambwa kwa'nanyembe*, the power of the knife, which has as its typical manifestation involuntary trembling at the sound of circumcision bells. His feelings of detachment from everyday life and concerns are thus linked to spiritual forces.

The other main point of interest is that this conversation took place early in the ritual cycle and while neither of the boys were dressed or dancing. Yet the boy clearly articulates, and in much the same way, themes that will be repeated over and over again to him later by elders in formal addresses. The boy clearly understands what is required of him and how he must prepare himself for the operation which entails a real, if remote, threat of death. The keynote is whole-hearted desire and steady concentration on the ordeal he faces. Such determination finds its natural expression in the dancing, and the tempo of the rites seems designed to gradually raise this to a pitch where the boy's single and overwhelming desire is to be cut.

The emphasis on self-determination gives a distinctive form to what in Van Gennep's scheme would be referred to as 'the rites of separation'. For example, a pattern common in the ethnographic literature is for such separation to be achieved by the abrupt and sometimes violent removal of the novices from the domestic setting, whence they are then taken to sacred sites of initiation in the bush to face unknown dangers. In such situations the novices appear relatively passive, submitting to the authority of the elders and initiated by them. Gisu separation rites display none of these features. In the first place, as has been made clear, the dangers which the boys face are known; second, the ceremonies are open, public events at all stages; third, they are regarded as neither secret nor esoteric. Nor, since the operations are performed in the domestic compound, is there any geographic separation of the candidate from his family and neighbours. Ritual separation is achieved rather through a succession of graduated steps, each one of which, significantly, is inaugurated by the boy himself. The emphasis is on his active preparation for the ordeal he faces.

The profile of the rites leading up to circumcision can be seen to mark three stages in the development of the candidate's commitment. The following description concentrates on the main types of activity in which the boy is involved and on features which are common throughout Bugisu.[11]

1   The circumcision year is ushered in during late January by the blowing of horns. From May until July individual candidates announce their intention of undergoing the ordeal by dressing in the special regalia and beginning to dance. The full regalia is extremely elaborate and flamboyant, with a head-dress made from the skin of a Colobus monkey and long tails decorated with cowrie shells which hang down his back and swirl in the dance. What items of costume a boy wears depends however on what he is lent by his kin or can hire or buy from others. The essentials are the

metal thigh bells, two or three to each leg, and strings of beads crossed over his chest. The individual items of costume are given no particular significance; it is the overall effect which is important. The costume is said to make the boy look 'wild'.

At this stage small groups of boys usually dance together, dancing along the paths and through the compounds of their neighbourhood, sometimes to assemble and display on an open space. The dancing at this time has a distinctive name and takes a stomping form unaccompanied by song. It is also sporadic. The period as a whole is known as *xuwetsa imbalu* – searching for *imbalu* – implying the gradual awakening of intent in the individual and its provisional nature. A boy may drop out at this stage without any disgrace.

2　The second phase begins in July, two or three weeks before the actual operation. It is marked by the boys threshing the millet which will be used to brew the beer which is offered to the ancestors and visitors on circumcision day. This is the first important ritual act and is taken as a clear sign of intent. It is accompanied by the sacrifice of a chicken and the inspection of its entrails. This is the first time that auguries are consulted for the boy.

Thereafter the dancing is known as *xusamba imbalu*, 'dancing *imbalu*', and is accompanied by song. Younger men and women as well as boys and girls now identify with particular candidates and accompany them on their travels. These are now more purposeful since the boy must visit all his close relatives and elicit their permission for the operation; that is, he must prove his fortitude through the strength of his dancing. These visits take a set form. The boy and his group dance into the compound, the closest relative then usually comes forward to address the boy, warns him of the ordeal he faces and urges that he dances with determination. One repeated theme of these speeches is that the boy must not confuse the glamour of his costume and the dance with *imbalu* itself. He is told that *imbalu* depends not on the costume but the person. Circumcision is not a game. He must think only of the ordeal he faces. The boy must remain silent under these often violently expressed tirades. He is then exhorted to show what he is worth by jumping. These jumps are regarded as extremely important and a good high jump is rewarded with a shout of encouragement. The jumps have the definite aspect of a test and are taken as indicative of his determination and how he will perform under the knife. Indeed, they can be seen as a direct rehearsal of the final jump the boy must make in the circumcision enclosure to show his readiness to face the circumcisers. Sacrifices or gifts are then offered to the boy and where he and his party have travelled a long way, and journeys of ten to twenty miles are not uncommon, they are feasted.

3   The third phase, which leads on directly to the operation itself, is again linked to the brewing of the circumcision beer. Two days before circumcision the boy pours water on the prepared millet and is then smeared from head to toe with millet yeast. From now until the operation in the afternoon of the third day all the important rituals to ensure the boy's ritual protection are concentrated. Sacrifices are offered for him by his mother's brother, his father's sister, and on the compound where he will stand the operation. For himself, his followers, his close kin and, where collective ceremonies are still performed, the lineage and sub-clans, the rites now involve a crescendo of activity and involvement.

Circumcision involves everybody and the atmosphere is charged with excitement. The boy himself dances more or less non-stop, the dances continuing often throughout the night as well as during the day. Emotions are running extremely high and circumcision dancing parties give way to no-one, with unwary passers-by risking getting a lash from the sticks they carry. For the boy, normal rules of conduct can appear suspended; his absorption in the dancing and thus in *imbalu* should be so total that the normal courtesies of everyday life are irrelevant. On circumcision day some boys appear to be in a trance-like state, though this trance is not that of 'possession', where the individual is not in control of his actions, but rather one induced by exclusive preoccupation with the ordeal he faces.[12]

The crescendo of involvement leading up to circumcision thus can be divided into a number of distinct phases. Each one is initiated by the candidate and marks not only his own increasing commitment to *imbalu* but mobilises those around him. At first the boy dances only intermittently, 'possible candidate' being only one aspect of his identity while his kin and others in the community are little more than passive bystanders. As the sequence progresses not only does the boy identify increasingly with *imbalu* but his relatives mobilise behind him until *imbalu* absorbs the attention of all. Throughout, the accent of responsibility never leaves the boy, for his actions are seen both to mark his commitment and precipitate the next ritual sequence. This stress on volition is apparent right up to the time of the operation itself. Where possible, the boy chooses the time of day that he will be cut and, even at the last, as he runs downhill towards the circumcision enclosure he is stopped by his mother's brother and asked if he is still firm. He may, even then, withdraw, otherwise he runs ahead into the enclosure to jump on the spot where protective medicines have been buried. The circumcisers, until then hidden, emerge and quickly perform the operation.

Volition, however important, is but one aspect. The energy put into the dancing and the aggressiveness of the circumcision parties are revealing of other important psychological and symbolic themes. Throughout the circumcision period the penis is referred to as *isolo* (the wild animal) and the overall effect of the boy's costume, as has been mentioned, is to make him 'look wild'.[13] With La Fontaine (1977), I would argue that this 'wildness' is far more than a convenient way of marking the dissociation from normal life typical of rites of separation. Since Van Gennep, we have grown accustomed to interpreting such rites as marking in a formal way the separation of the novice from the community, the sacred from the profane. Separation then has been viewed more as a state than as an active process with important psychological concomitants. However, La Fontaine writes that, for the Gisu, the period called 'dancing the circumcision' is a purposeful activity which is aimed not just at setting the novices apart but at increasing their strength. This strength is now linked to the development of *lirima* in the boys.[14]

The key feature of *lirima* is the intensity of the emotion experienced. It is further seen as uncontrollable, being said to 'bubble-up' in a man, or perhaps 'boil over', since the usual simile is with the boiling of milk. Attribution of *lirima* thus implies that a man is completely in the grip of the particular emotion. It 'catches' him, 'bubbles up' in him and, while in that state of possession, it dictates his actions and attitudes. Jealousy, hatred, anger, resentment – for all of which there are Gisu words – may inspire such violent effect. One might add, in parenthesis, that the situations in which it is adduced and its breadth of reference make it tempting to equate *lirima* with a state of sympathetic arousal of the nervous system, an equation made the more plausible by the fact that the Gisu associated *lirima* and, indeed, sometimes define it with the sensation of having a lump in the throat. Such a symptom could well be produced by the release of adrenalin and the subsequent contraction of the muscles of the throat.[15]

In normal life it is the capacity of men, and only men, for *lirima* that marks them out as dangerous; *lirima*, indeed, having generally negative connotations and being associated with violence. A good man is thus one whose *lirima* is strictly under control and who is thus slow to anger.

18

'Goodness' in this sense is seen as a dispositional attribute of a person and associated as mentioned earlier with the heart. In this context, the first washing of the boy by the circumciser on the morning following the operation is revealing. This is the only occasion on which he is given any formal teaching or instruction on his new role and he is bound solely by moral injunctions. After cleansing the boy's hands, the circumciser gives him food, fire, a hoe, a knife, a drinking tube and other utensils of adult life. As each item is handed to him the boy is told both of its proper use and of its misuse, for example, 'Kindle this piece of firewood and as you kindle it I say, "Do not go and burn down the houses of your neighbours. I have made you kindle it so that your wife can cook for you and you can heat water and make tea for yourselves" … I give you this drinking tube to hold and say, "Drink beer and brew it. Do not get drunk and quarrelsome so that you are always fighting with your friends"' … and so on. The context makes it clear that this is not only a form of teaching through contrasts, though it is this, but is linked to the ambivalent qualities of manhood. The Gisu boy is entering into a world of relatively free competition with other men. *Lirima* might be essential, on the one hand, for the independent assertiveness required of Gisu men but, on the other, it has its natural outlet in violent retributive action.

What must be stressed is that this ambivalence of *lirima* is a basic fact of life; it is not something which can be tampered with or altered. It is inherent in the nature of men. And, central to the transformational process of *imbalu* is that this is the first time in which the boy is expected to display the emotion. Indeed, it is induced for the first time at *imbalu*. Thereafter it is as much a part of his manhood as the circumcision cut itself. Moreover, in the context of circumcision, *lirima* is accorded a positive and essential role. For the Gisu it is the key to the complete identification of the boy with the ordeal he faces. As the ordeal gets closer it is *lirima* which drives him on and dominates his thoughts and feelings.

In her account of the Bemba *chisungu*, Richards notes that the relatively minor ordeals of the jumping tests tended to be mentioned in even the most abbreviated accounts of the ritual and excited most interest, indeed anxiety, in actual performance. Such tests were linked by the Bemba both to the idea of the rites as 'making the girl grow' and to 'teaching her'. The element of formal teaching of new responsibilities, Richards notes, was minimal, and even then, superfluous, since all girls were familiar with the duties and privileges of adulthood. Nor was there much attempt to instruct the girl on the occasion of her *chisungu* on the mysteries of the ritual symbols so carefully constructed by the women in charge. Covered by blankets and secluded in a corner of the hut the girl was often in a poor position to see anything. Rather, the teaching occurred at another level and was more a matter of teaching the correct attitudes towards experience which prepare the girl for 'the transition from a calm but unproductive girlhood to a potentially dangerous but fertile womanhood' (Richards, 1956a: 125). In such a context the tests appear as tangible proofs both to herself and to others that 'she is actually a "grown-up" and can safely and successfully behave like one' (ibid.: 162).

The acquisition of new powers and proof of the attainment of these is even more crucial for Gisu *imbalu*. At the beginning many boys evidence doubt and apprehension as to their ability to withstand the ordeal. One way of looking at the ritual sequence and how it works to effect a change of attitudes would be to say that in the course of the rituals the boy is made to identify with the attitudes and emotions of adult men – he must present himself as a fully responsible agent freely choosing the ordeal and sticking to this resolution. From this point of view one could argue that volition and *lirima* are key themes in the ritual because they constitute what it is to be a man. Through identification with these, and the constant testing for such qualities, the boy learns in the course of the ritual to experience himself and his potentialities differently, as a man rather than as a boy. Enduring the operation is thus the final proof that such a transformational process is complete.[16]

Such an interpretation can never be more than a partial gloss on the process. In order to probe deeper into Gisu idiom and the power they impute to their ritual forms, attention must be turned to the last three days of the ritual in which are concentrated the rites which finally strengthen the boy for the ordeal. In explicating the symbolism of these rites the emphasis on the preparation of the boy for the ordeal will be given priority. Indeed, the claim is made that much of this symbolism is only explicable with regard to the concern with psychological utility – what Richards called 'pragmatic effects', rather than, for example, with regard to the presentation of social values, especially when these are narrowly interpreted in terms of principles of social organisation.

The rites of fortification

The emotional pitch of the culminating phase of the rituals, which begins with the boy pouring water on his beer and ends with the operation, has already been commented upon. These three days stand out from the previous phases in other ways as well: activity is not only more intense but is also imbued with a potency that is missing from the previous rites. Certain things, especially those which signal a lack of physical control, are held not only to be unpropitious but mystically dangerous for the boy. This applies to stumbling or falling and in some cases a sacrifice must be made to avert the danger. The boy is now seen as entering an extremely dangerous state and for the first time is brought into the orbit of powers beyond his direct control which may affect his success not only at the time of the operation, but also his ability to heal and, indeed, the entire course of his life thereafter. The sacrifices made at this time have the overt aim of protecting the boy against the dangers of witchcraft and cursing by his senior kinsmen and to insure against any retributive intervention by the ancestral ghosts, all factors which are held to be capable of causing a prolonged and painful healing process, or lead to his failure in adult life.[17] In the present context, however, the more interesting rites are those which have the explicit aim not of protecting the boy from evil influences but of directly fortifying him for the ordeal.

During the three days leading up to the operation the boy is successively smeared with three substances: yeast, chyme (see below) and, in the areas of the South and Central Bugisu where collective, lineage-based rituals are still held, black swamp mud.[18]

The yeast-smearing rite is known as *cimolo* and is first performed immediately after the boy has poured water on the millet for his circumcision beer, that is, on the morning of the third day before circumcision. Later on that same day his mother will add millet yeast (*kamamera*) to the brew, thus beginning the final fermentation. This millet yeast is made from germinated finger millet seed which is then ground to powder. Some of the powder from this batch is mixed with water to form a thick paste which the smearing elder uses to cover the boy completely from head to toe. This elder is a senior agnate, chosen explicitly because of his own bravery at circumcision. Ideally the boy stands for this rite on the place in the compound where he will actually stand for the operation. The *cimolo* rite is repeated on each of three days leading up to circumcision and the thick encrustation of dried yeast gives the boy a distinctive appearance.

In addition to the yeast the boy is usually smeared twice with chyme, *buse*, from the stomach of sacrificial goats. Sacrifice is offered first by the mother's brother to ensure the protection of the maternal ancestors and may take place on any of the three days. A second sacrifice, this time for the paternal ancestors, takes place on the morning of circumcision day in the compound where the boy will stand for the operation. After both these sacrifices chyme is smeared on the boy in patches, on the forehead, cheeks, chest, stomach and limbs, thus overlaying the yeast. The first smearing is done by the mother's brother, the second by the elder who smeared the boy with yeast.

Unlike the smearing with yeast and chyme, the smearing with mud does not take place in the domestic setting but at special mudding swamps associated with the *kumusambwa kw'imbalu* and reserved for this purpose alone. Early on the morning of circumcision the elders of the swamp sacrifice a chicken and pour a libation of beer on the site. They then literally prepare the ground by stamping on it until it forms a foaming mire. The boys arrive late in the afternoon. Typically, in the areas where lineage-based rituals are held, the boy leaves the compound around mid-morning after being smeared with yeast and chyme. He then takes an individually devised route, designed to avoid major paths where sorcery substances are feared and to lead him to the houses of his closest relatives and from these to the communal dancing ground, where he and his party will meet up with other circumcision parties in the mid-afternoon. From there the parties set off first for the ancestral grove (*icirindwa*) where the boys are collectively blessed by the elders of the area by the blowing of beer over them. From there they proceed to the swamps. Here the elder of the swamp blesses them individually with beer and, depending on the depth of the swamp, they then either jump in or stand on the side while the elder smears them all over with the black mud. The boys then return directly back to their separate compounds for the operation.

Each of these smearings is accompanied by exhortations to the boy of a very similar kind. In content the speeches are more specific and precise than the tirades from seniors that I have mentioned so far. The atmosphere is also different. The smearing elder does not have to shout amid the hubbub to get his voice heard, for the smearing rites are events of great solemnity and the bystanders fall silent. The elder's speech is slow, deliberate and emphatic. He now gives the final advice and instructions on how the boy should stand for the operation and impresses upon him that *imbalu* is a 'tough' or 'fierce' thing; he must understand it at this level and make sure he has the strength to go through with it. The smearing rite brings the boy to the brink of circumcision itself and concern with how the boy will react under the knife is paramount. He must stand for the smearing as he should do for *imbalu* – upright, staring fixedly in front of him, taking this comparatively minor abuse of his body stoically. It can be noted that in the normal course of events this kind of smearing would be regarded as abhorrent and extremely unpleasant, and some boys smile in embarrassment when first being smeared in this fashion. Later the boy becomes used to the experience and such a sign of levity is unthinkable at the mud-smearing stage. The smearing rite itself also yields other clues as to the determination of the boy – particularly the 'jumps' with which it ends and which should be done with extreme vigour. The important concern continues to be whether the boy's heart is really in it, whether he has *imbalu* in him (*imbalu ilimo*), or whether he is still simply making a show of intent.

If one asks how the Gisu themselves conceive the smearing of substances as working to affect the psychological state of the boy, then it appears on the basis of the evidence presented so far that they could be seen simply as a dramatic and forceful reiteration of the themes so far outlined as characteristic of the ritual. Thus, the locus of responsibility rests squarely with the boy, and any efficacy attributed to the smearing substances rests on their power to impress the boy yet again with the nature of the undertaking. One strand of Gisu exegetical tradition does indeed account for the smearing rites in such terms:

> They smear the boy with all these things to see if he is intent on circumcision. They make his whole body cold so that he shivers and is covered with goosepimples. The yeast shows him that he must be a tough man. They show him that *imbalu* is tough and he goes knowing that *imbalu* is tough…. These things make him cold and shivery. Mud, chyme and yeast dry out the boy's skin. He feels them gripping his skin. They show him that he too must be fierce and determined and he knows that he is going for circumcision. Circumcision is fierce and these things with which they smear him give him strength. They are done for the strength of the *kumusambwa kw'imbalu* (ancestral power of *imbalu*). People do these things in order to change him into a very fierce person, different from others. He is like another person. He has only the intention to think about *imbalu*. He feels that his body is cold and so these things show him fierceness. And when they make him jump they encourage him saying '*ingi, ingi, ingi!*' And when he jumps high and low with vigour it shows that he is really fierce. You go to war and fight with all your strength. You must make yourself see that you have enough strength to overcome another man's strength. So these things are like being prepared for war.

This text, reproduced verbatim, was given to me by an elder in Central Bugisu and is an extremely common mode of interpretation, similar views being reported by Turner (1969). One point of interest here is that it is perfectly compatible with the symbolic/expressive interpretation of ritual, most associated with Beattie, where the efficacy of ritual is argued to lie in the power of dramatic expression, through the acting out of 'what is sought, and held important, to say' (Beattie, 1966: 68). One of the objections to this view of the ritual process is that it tends to set up a polarity between observers' and participants' accounts, the former talking about ritual in terms of its ability to communicate values and shape the attitudes of the participants, while the latter apparently intend their ritual to influence spiritual powers and thus achieve ends beyond normal human compass.[19] In the Gisu text above there is, however, no such tension, for the emphasis is on the facility of yeast and the other smearing substances through their glutinous properties and the way they dry on the skin to represent to the boy the idea of 'fierceness'. It is not implied that any magical potency is inherent in the yeast itself; rather, if the yeast has power it is because it provides an external representation of a desired internal orientation. Other verbal analogies play on the same idea, the boy must 'hold tight' to *imbalu* in the same way as the yeast 'holds tight' to his skin. Moreover, the smearings are seen here to be very much like the 'telling', both words and actions convey the same message. It is pertinent to note here that very little is said directly about the smearing substances during the rite. The most common form of reference usually occurs in the form 'As I smear you with yeast I say, "Be firm for *imbalu*".' Thus, although the yeast is definitely associated with firmness, I never heard it said that the yeast *will* make you firm for *imbalu*. The same goes for the speeches made in conjunction with the smearings of chyme and mud; they are exhortations to the boy, and seemingly carry none of the efficacy or character of, for example, a spell.

From this perspective the smearing rites act as yet another mnemonic to the boy designed to inculcate the necessary determination. Other aspects of the ritual situation reinforce and elaborate upon the same message: the elders' speeches, the mortification of the smearings foretelling the further mortification to come and, lastly, his body encrusted with yeast as a clear sign to himself and others that he is finally 'set apart' and so set upon his course. Direct psychological efficacy without the mediation of spiritual powers is implied in other Gisu interpretations of the smearing rites as well. Humiliation is sometimes given as the purpose of the rites. Thus I was told that they are done 'to punish' the boy, the term 'punish' here carrying not the implication of a punishment for an offence committed but rather the idea of mortification. This it is implied will anger him, incite his *lirima*, and thus spur him on. This is a slightly more complex account solely because it depends upon knowing the kinds of emotional effects the Gisu desire, and how this relates to the aim of changing him into 'a very fierce person, different from others'.

The idea of the yeast as gripping the skin as a physical embodiment of fierceness, toughness and determination is not, however, the only mode of Gisu exegesis. What, from one point of view, is symbolism and mimesis is, from another, metaphysical power, and the two strands mingle easily in Gisu thought. The same elder whom I quoted above, and who was in no sense a ritual specialist though possibly an exceptionally articulate elder, also gave another interpretation which sheds a different light on the smearing substances. It brings in the idea of a magical interchange of properties between the substances and the boy:

> These things, mud, chyme, yeast and beer are all mixed up and in this they are alike. They are like the mud in that it is the soil which they have stamped on and walked on so they have mixed it with water from below to form mud. When it bubbles it erupts like porridge. They say that the kumusambwa *kw'imbalu* is there, for even if it is dry the mud there bubbles by itself without rain and looks as though someone has brewed beer. We say that the *kumusambwa* has brewed its beer. That mud is its beer and when it bubbles they say it has fermented. And then the boys must jump in that mud and return to be circumcised. They have jumped in the beer of the *kumusambwa kw'imbalu*.

This constitutes an extended metaphor which can be taken in a number of directions, the most important of which is that the substances are alike in that they are 'mixed up' and ultimately like beer: that is, in a state of fermentation, activity and change. This is clearly linked to the presence of the ancestral powers and the boy's last act is to jump into the mud – the 'beer' created by the *kumusambwa kw'imbalu*. The first aspect to look at, therefore, is the ritual significance of beer and the kinds of concordance drawn between the boy, the process of fermentation and the ancestral powers.

The prestigious finger millet beer, *busera*, which is used for all rituals, takes two to three weeks to make and involves two distinct periods of fermentation. The first fermentation is used to give colour and flavour to the brew and is achieved by dampening millet flour with water and leaving it covered in a dark place for about a week. Any alcohol and yeast are then removed by roasting this millet porridge over a fierce heat. Water and fresh millet yeast are then added to produce a second fermentation, with the beer drunk on the third day. At circumcision the boy initiates both these fermentations, the first by threshing the millet, the second by pouring water on the roasted porridge. As beer is regarded as essential for all rituals, many of them are geared to the second three-day beer brewing cycle, but in no other is the person at the centre of the ritual involved in its preparation. The participation of the boy at circumcision draws attention to and effectively synchronises two processes: the growth of his determination and the fermentation of beer. Thus the beer-brewing cycle is doing far more than simply orchestrating the sequence of the rites; it also reflects in a fundamental way on the nature of the boy's commitment. Hence, it is significant that the second fermentation should be quick and active, the brew clearly 'bubbling-up' (*xatubana*). This fermentation is always associated with the ancestors and is likewise indicative of *lirima*. Thus it is said that the effervescence shows that both the ancestors and *lirima* are in the beer. The boy and the beer are thus similarly held to be imbued with ancestral power and *lirima*.

The form of the rituals, the text quoted and the associations of beer and *lirima* make it clear that real analogies are drawn between the boy and the beer. The two are brought into further direct association through the smearing rites, since the smearing substances all gain their significance through their association with beer; the yeast as the initiator of fermentation, the chyme and the mud because of their eruptive qualities. At this point, we might ask whether the identification of the boy and the beer is simply a basic metaphor, conceptually illuminating some of the aspects of change, or whether the ritual is believed to effect an active transference of properties, not only identifying the boy with fermenting things, but intended to induce such 'ferment' in himself. Potency, as Ahern (1979) has pointed out, is not a uniform property of ritual acts, and belief takes a variety of different forms. As has been seen, the Gisu do offer interpretations of the smearing rites which are basically naturalistic and do not involve ideas of metaphysical transformation. Moreover, many other aspects of the ritual are clearly 'symbolic' in the sense of signifying or making statements without these being believed to have any power to achieve the desired ends in themselves. A case in point is the boy's costume. Dressing in the costume signifies the boy's intent, but he is explicitly warned against falling into the fallacy of assuming that it will directly get him through the ordeal. He is told '*imbalu* is not the costume but the person'. Apart from its signifying and orientating function, what power the costume has is of a metaphoric kind, connecting ideas which are then capable of extension, thus widening the sphere of reference in a reflexive way.[20] Specifically, the costume draws attention to the associations: penis/boy/wild animal/ancestors, which open up in an evocative way different possibilities for reflecting on the nature of the transition in which the boy is involved. Such possibilities may or may not be exploited.

But the smearing rites are not metaphoric in this way alone. In the first place, they are undoubtedly considered to be powerful in themselves. The importance attached to the smearing rites, the magical charge of the last three days and the fact that even the bravery of the smearing elder is held to have a direct effect on the fortitude of the boy, support the idea that the smearing substances are believed to have the power to not only represent qualities but actually impart them. Second, it appears that the figurative power of the rites is to this end restricted. Metaphor, as it is involved here, is 'a device for seeing something in terms of something else' (Burke, 1945: 503), and where metaphors are put to use in this way the relevant analogy must be salient. One concept, then, tends to give coherence to the symbolic field and it is through this that the rites are seen to achieve their end.[21] In the course of the smearing rites the boy is brought into a relationship, and progressively identified, with the ancestral powers and other potent things 'fermenting' with *lirima*. The smearing rites thus encapsulate and advance the process of change in which the boy is involved.

Gisu exegesis on the subject of how their rituals work gives the lie to Mauss' adage that people are always content to know how to perform rituals and have little speculative interest in their 'mechanics' (Mauss, 1972: 56). Two different Gisu interpretations of the smearing rites have been outlined above. While both are seen to impart fortitude they can be seen to do so in different ways, one of which can be broadly classed as 'realist', with ultimate efficacy resting on the intervention of spiritual powers and the potency of objects, the other can be classed as 'symbolic' in so far as it tends to put the stress on the power of objects to show and demonstrate aims and attitudes. They also exploit a different, though overlapping, range of ideas. More significantly perhaps, the locus of responsibility is altered from one version to the other. Where the sensation of the yeast on the skin alone is deemed efficacious the onus remains firmly on the boy to identify himself with the desired end – the substances 'show him that he too must be fierce and determined and he knows that he is going for circumcision'. But, in the alternative version, the boy is only one agent in a field of interacting forces, each of which is held powerful without the boy's conscious identification. In the actual situation of the smearing rites both these aspects are implicated and so these different accounts could be said to pose, but not resolve, the basic tension which exists in Gisu thought between the stress on the idea of the boy being in control of his own fate as opposed to ideas that he is subject to external influences beyond his control.[22]

Creative powers, *lirima* and manhood

In the last section it has been seen that the smearing rites have an explicit psychological aim, directed towards making the boy 'tough', 'fierce' and different from others in terms of such qualities. Moreover, it is also evident that Gisu have a lively interest in, and a number of ways of explaining, how their rituals achieve this intended effect. The 'fermentation model' outlined above adds a significant new dimension to our understanding of how the process is conceived. In the light of it we can perhaps read more into the ordering of the smearing triad. One possible interpretation might be that the yeast initiates the process of fermentation, the chyme presents the process of active conversion (in the stomach of an animal) and the mud, as the beer of the ancestral power of *imbalu*, presents fermentation as the end in itself. So, too, the awakening, growth and culmination of *lirima* in the boy. *Lirima* is induced with the specific aim of allowing the boy to stand the ordeal.

Lirima and fermentation are seen to share a number of characteristics: both are volatile, 'strong', 'bitter' and 'potent'. Moreover, where previously *lirima* has been described in conjunction with the emotions, it now seems more appropriate to see it as a type of 'power' or an aspect of creative energy. Indeed, through its association with fermentation, it is presented as one of the creative processes in the cosmos, on a par with human procreation.

The model used by the Gisu to understand human fertility is not taken from analogy with seeds and vegetable fertility but is rather the process of fermentation. In procreation it is believed that the 'white blood' (semen) of a man mixes together with the 'red blood' (placental) of a woman to form a child. The substance of the child is thus deemed to be equally formed from male and female fluids, and frequent intercourse during the first six months of pregnancy is thought necessary to develop a healthy foetus. As in beer fermentation, the 'bloods' inside the woman are said to 'bubble up' and this volatility of gestation is considered liable to spill over and affect the woman emotionally. Again, 'bubbling-up' carries the overtones of *lirima*, and this fermentation model of gestation is used to explain a number of the characteristics of pregnancy. For women, it is seen as a time of heightened emotion, of irritability and bad temper. Further, in terms of the parallelism with fermentation, gestation also has a spiritual counterpart, indicative of the presence of the ancestral spirits with the child inheriting at birth the life force of someone in his kindred who has recently died.

With fermentation as the linking model, both procreation and the transformation of the boy in *imbalu* can be seen as exemplifying a similar form of creative energy and can be explicitly compared as processes.[23] One could perhaps say that as the creative power of women manifests itself in childbirth, so the creative power of men manifests itself in circumcision and that of beer in fermentation. Additionally, the act of circumcision, as La Fontaine (1971) makes clear, creates a number of different ways of commenting upon the relative powers of the sexes. The complex potentialities inherent here can be indicated by the fact that the cuts of circumcision can be compared in terms of pain with childbirth, while in terms of blood loss, parallels can be drawn with defloration, menstruation and the blood of parturition. Since the Gisu exploit the full range here, many different themes can be discerned and their implications traced to a number of diverse and not necessarily consistent conclusions. However, the cognised model most relevant in the context of the rituals is that circumcision creates a specifically male power.

The most common myth associated with circumcision tells in a straightforward way how the practice originated through the marriage of a Gisu man with a woman from one of the Nandi-speaking peoples whose territory borders that of the Gisu. Nandi women practise clitoridectomy, but when the woman cut her daughters the men saw that this made them 'too strong' and so began cutting themselves instead. Such 'strength' could, as mentioned before, be translated as strength of character. For the Gisu it is related to *lirima* which is seen to give force to volition so that it is carried through to completion. It is the ability to act resolutely, to carry through projects to their conclusion which in general distinguishes *lirima* from the weaker arousal of *libuba* experienced by women and children. *Lirima* thus underlies the major distinction between the sexes and their potentialities. Men are by definition more powerful than women, they have greater authority (*bunyala*) and greater physical strength (*kamani*). But the attribute of *lirima* gives yet another dimension to maleness, for it is also tied to the negative emotions – hatred, anger and vengeance.

Here, it is important to stress again the creative power of the ritual. Before circumcision boys are held to be incapable of *lirima*, and for this reason their misdemeanours are usually discounted. Revealing of Gisu attitudes on this score is an exceptional case where there was strong body of local feeling that a youth of about sixteen who had gained a reputation for aggressive trouble-making should be killed. Many others, however, held equally firmly that the killing of children was a senseless act since by definition the weaker powers of a child could pose no serious threat to adult interests. In such terms child-killing is an abomination. The counter argument was, however, that evidence of such an anti-social disposition in one so young boded extremely ill for the future. After circumcision this tendency could only be intensified and his *lirima* would be put to ever more violent ends. The significance of this case is to show not only that *lirima* as a concept has strong explanatory power in everyday discourse about the nature of the personality but that the transforming effect of circumcision has for the Gisu a real and not just a formal dimension. A boy takes on not just the mantle and responsibilities of adulthood but becomes a man with the distinctive capacities of a man. That male force to act on and in the world carries the threat of violence is for the Gisu an evident, but unquestioned, cost of their collective identity.

At the most evident level the rites dramatically assert the unity of male experience. Boys are initiated and become men in exactly the same way as their seniors and are heirs to the same status in the community. 'Let the son resemble his father' is the chorus line of one of the most popular circumcision songs. From this perspective, it is the aspect of continuity which comes to the fore: the boys simultaneously prove that they are equal to their seniors and to the generations before them and in so doing they demonstrate the continued strength of the *kumusambwa kw'imbalu*. To reiterate, this is seen as directly catching the initiates with the desire to take circumcision. The potency of *imbalu* as a cultural symbol rests on this aspect: the linked ancestry of all Gisu and the continuation of the powers which go with it.

The vernacular psychology of ritual

At the beginning of this chapter, it was argued that the nature of circumcision as a culturally focal symbol could not be explicated simply by looking at its politico-jural implications or by seeing how social roles and relationships are transfigured in the ritual. Instead, it was argued that one needed a different kind of input, and one which took more seriously the claim of such rites actively to transform the individual. This has involved a focus on what might be called the 'vernacular psychology' of the rites, seeing this as informing the overall sequence of the ritual and being given emphatic expression in the symbolism.

This opens up the question of how far ritual forms are constrained or determined by their psychological goals rather than by their ability to codify and express the social structure. In fact, the issue is not one of choice between these alternatives but of their relative priority, as Victor Turner's exploratory work on the psychological dimensions of ritual has demonstrated.[24] Instead of immediate recourse to depth or any other western psychology I would, however, argue for an initial consideration in participant terms, thus allowing any overt psychological themes to become apparent. The contribution of the communicative aspects of ritual symbols, then, is not to carry largely hidden messages about social relations but to directly structure the psychological field in which the individual is prepared and made capable of acting.

The distinctive character of Gisu circumcision rituals can in these terms be ascribed to the dual emphasis on volition and *lirima*. Throughout, the boy is seen as freely submitting himself to the ordeal and this resolution is tied to the growth of *lirima* within him. And what from one point of view is preparation of the boy for the ordeal is, from another, its culmination. The induction of *lirima* thus appears both as a technique of the ritual, induced in the boy to allow him to stand the ordeal, and also its aim, to turn him into a man, with the capacity thereafter to feel *lirima*.

This chapter has not been concerned to explicate all the idioms of Gisu vernacular psychology relevant to *imbalu* – that would be an enormous task. By concentrating on the major themes, the aim has been to show that the Gisu have a set of psychological, as well as religious, concepts which inform their actions in the ritual. Moreover, the psychological processes built into the ritual clearly 'work' in the sense that they provide the means which enable often extremely apprehensive boys to overcome their fear and stand the ordeal. Quantitative measures are difficult here, but I would estimate that at least seven or eight boys out of ten succeed completely in displaying the required fortitude under the knife. Of the rest, some evade the ordeal by having the operation in hospital or going secretly to circumcisers believed to administer an anaesthetic, and a few break down or show some sign of fear at the end. Given the success of the rites in these terms, the question arises as to whether the psychological process and concepts, such as *lirima*, answer solely to the culturally specific Gisu construction of experience or whether they answer also to a universal experiential base. Given our limited knowledge of psychological processes, enquiry into this latter area can perhaps be seen to involve little more than a process of translation, a seeking of concordances between the terms of vernacular and western psychologies. Despite its difficulties, this would seem to be one of the most exciting areas for the further exploration and understanding of ritual forms.

3

THE RITUAL USE OF VIOLENCE

Circumcision among the Gisu of Uganda

There has been considerable recent interest in the subjective effects of
ordeals and initiations, with writers concerned not only to elaborate
upon the ideas mediated through the ritual process but also to speculate upon the effects of the experience on the individual. This chapter
looks at a ritual which may be said to use violence to achieve violence
– the circumcision ritual among the Gisu of Uganda. My initial
concerns are with the kind of sense that may be given to the Gisu view
that a capacity for being violent is engendered – indeed created –
through the circumcision experience. How should we begin to understand the psychological processes involved?

Gisu boys are circumcised when they are between eighteen and
twenty-five years old, and the practice effectively denotes their sense of
ethnic identity and distinctiveness (see Chapters One and Nine of this
volume and La Fontaine, 1969 and Twaddle, 1969). It is the only major
ritual observance shared by all. Circumcision is also a classic-type
ordeal, an explicit test of bravery publicly witnessed. The boy stands in
the compound of his father or senior relative and must remain absolutely still while his foreskin is cut and then stripped from around the
glans penis. He is required to display total fortitude under the knife,
betraying no signs of fear; even what might be regarded as involuntary
twitches and tremblings, such as the blinking of the eyes, are evaluated
negatively. Success, however, is triumphantly celebrated; the watching
men roar in unison while the women rush forward ululating as they
dance. The boy is then allowed to sit and the onlookers come forward one
by one to call him a man and to thank him by presenting him with gifts.

Undergoing the ordeal makes a boy (*umusinde*) a 'man', and the
honorific term *umusani* is always used in this context. This is an
acknowledgement of the achievement of manhood, for the term is
usually reserved for men who have proved themselves through having
adult children, especially circumcised sons. In the success of the ordeal,

it is used to address both the son and his father. In other respects, too, circumcision gives the son a formal identity with his father since it gives him full adult status, carrying with it the all-important rights to marry, to inherit land and to enjoy such other privileges of adult life as drinking beer.

In the previous chapter, it was argued that the ritual can be understood to do far more than formally bequeath status. Undergoing the ordeal is regarded by the Gisu as having a basic effect on the personality and powers of the individual. The ritual thus has a definite ontological purpose; it is seen to create in the boy the capacity to experience *lirima*, and it is this capacity which critically marks the divide between boys and men.

Lirima is pre-eminently a manly quality. There is no easy equivalent in English. One might start with the idea that it refers to violent emotion, and many of the ways in which the Gisu talk about it suggest that such emotion is also experienced as overwhelming and even out-of-control. Thus *lirima* is spoken of as 'catching' a man and as 'bubbling-up' in him – though 'boiling over' might be more appropriate as the usual simile is with the boiling of milk. While a man is in this state of possession, *lirima* is seen to dictate his attitudes and actions; it gives force to his motivations and impels him to action. Further, *lirima* is linked to the negative emotions, especially to anger, but also to jealousy, hatred, resentment and shame (the Gisu have an extensive vocabulary for such emotions), which are also seen as capable of inspiring such violent effects.

One could add, though tentatively and bearing in mind the difficulties of directly linking emotions to physiological stimuli (Schacter and Singer, 1962), that it is tempting to associate *lirima* with a state of sympathetic arousal of the nervous system, considering the situations in which it is adduced and its breadth of reference. This equation is made more plausible by the fact that the Gisu associate *lirima*, and indeed sometimes define it, with the sensation of having a lump in the throat. Such a symptom could well be produced by the release of adrenalin and the subsequent contraction of the muscles of the throat. While this possibly points to a certain parallelism between the Gisu concept and our own model (or one of them) for understanding intense or extreme emotions, one must be wary of any easy equivalence at this point. At issue is not just the indeterminacy of the (or indeed, any) physiological input in relation to the experience of emotion, but the cognitive associations which set the Western and Gisu models at variance.[1] For example, in Western conceptions, such extreme effect tends to suggest the overriding of reason by passion – a lack of self-control. In contrast, for the Gisu, who do not think of reason and emotion as opposed modalities embattled within the personality, *lirima* can not only be volitional but also an aspect of the control a man should assert over himself and the world – a quality or capacity to be mustered by the individual to achieve and serve his purposes. If a man can be in the grip of *lirima* he can use it to steel himself too. Then, *lirima* also has forceful and positive connotations; the force that lies behind that strength of character which makes men coura-geous and determined. That *lirima* bestows such affirmative powers, and is a capacity of men and only men, gives overall poignancy to its more usual associations. In normal, everyday life *lirima* is seen to have generally negative effects. It makes men dangerous and is asso-ciated with violence, aggression and the disorders which assail the community.

It can be noted here, since it forms part of the problem to be addressed, that the Gisu have long had a reputation for violence in East Africa. In Uganda they are widely feared for their personal aggressiveness. In the 1950s, Richards indicated the attitude of the Ganda towards those Gisu who had taken up settlement in their homeland: 'Ganda just steal but Gisu come with knives and kill you' (Richards, 1956b: 116). In Kenya their reputation is more lurid since they are proverbially regarded as cannibals – cannibalism indeed often being defined with reference to the Gisu. Even within Bugisu this reputation clings to certain clans. That the attribution of violence is not solely a matter of negative 'outsider' definitions is indicated by crime statistics which do indicate relatively high rates of interpersonal violence. Again the pattern is consistent. In the 1940s and 1950s, the Gisu had a homicide rate of 8.2 deaths per 100,000 people, higher than any of the other Bantu-speaking peoples of Uganda (Southall, 1960a: 228). In the 1960s, the differential was even more striking, with the Ugandan Police figures indicating a rate of 28.4 per 100,000 for Bugisu in 1963, over twice that of any other Bantu-speaking group.[2] It must be emphasised that this killing is almost entirely of an interpersonal kind: there is no raiding, feuding or warfare pattern. Further, it is overwhelmingly male/male, with women only forming 16.7 per cent of the victims and entering the statistics as killers even less frequently – in only 3.6 per cent of cases. The Gisu are cogniscent of this situation and it is not one of which they feel proud. One feature is an almost fatalistic acceptance of violence in the community. After a murder a commonly voiced sentiment was not just that the killer was a bad man but that the

Gisu were just bad people and what could one do? This capacity for violence is attributed to *lirima*.

What must be stressed is that, for the Gisu, the ambivalence of *lirima* is a basic fact of life and regarded as inherent in the nature of men. It is central to the transformational purpose of circumcision, for this is the first time at which the boy is expected to display the emotion. Thereafter it is as much a part of his manhood as the circumcision cuts themselves. Moreover, in the context of circumcision, *lirima* is accorded a positive and essential role. For the Gisu it is the key to the complete identification of the boy with the ordeal he faces. As the ordeal gets closer it is *lirima* which is seen to drive him on and to dominate his thoughts and feelings. It is *lirima* which allows him to overcome his fear. The induction of *lirima* thus appears both as a technique of the ritual, developed in the boy to allow him to stand the ordeal, and also its aim, to turn him into a man with the capacity thereafter to feel *lirima*.

In the last chapter I was concerned to explore the degree to which the ritual leading up to the operation itself – its form and symbolism – could be interpreted from the point of view of its overt aim, to induce *lirima*. Thus, I argued that the symbolic forms were best explicated not in the latent terms of the standard sociological version as making largely hidden statements about social relationships, but in terms of their manifest purpose – the making of men out of boys in the specifically Gisu way. Thus the rites have an overt transformational aim, a psychological purpose, and this could be described in terms of what I called Gisu vernacular psychology. Further, I felt that the rites and the psychological processes built into them clearly 'worked' – in the sense that they provided the means which enabled often extremely apprehensive boys to overcome their fear and stand the ordeal. Success here is never assured but I would estimate that the majority, say seven to eight out of ten, succeeded in displaying the required fortitude.

The ritual, then, can be seen to have pragmatic aims and pragmatic effects. This leads me to my next set of problems and a much more tricky set, given – as Audrey Richards (1967) once noted – that British social anthropology is littered with self-denying ordinances, especially on questions which might have anything to do with the individual experience or individual psychology. In brief, my problems revolve around the following query. If the rites can be seen to be informed by Gisu vernacular psychology and be seen to 'work' in these terms, can they also be seen to *work* in our psychological terms? Do concepts such as *lirima*, and the techniques used to induce it, answer solely to the culturally specific Gisu construction of experience, or can they also be seen to answer to a universal experiential base?

Clearly this cannot be easily answered given that neither anthropology nor psychology has given us any way of establishing universal processes and constraints. The only way of proceeding, I would argue, is in terms of a process of translation – of a seeking of concordances between the models given by vernacular and Western psychologies. Elucidation can then proceed by a to-ing and fro-ing between what Geertz (1983) refers to as 'experience-near' and 'experience-distant' concepts, by which different forms of local knowledge may be rendered mutually intelligible. One implication of this approach is that 'our' concepts, except in so far as they are the way 'we' explicate the world, may initially be accorded no specially privileged status. If we seek to translate, it is because we desire to perceive the analogies – not because of an assumption that our discourse, whether scientific or not, necessarily leads to a better way of construing the original.

The role of violence in ritual revolves around the emotional effects of ritual more generally. As an anthropologist, one has to admit, with Gluckman (1964), that one is here quickly 'beyond one's sphere of competence'. Yet this cannot legislate against curiosity, especially when emotional arousal is the cornerstone of the Durkheimian theory of ritual, alone accounting for the power attributed to ritual symbols and their ability to reinforce social values. Yet, when Leach (1958) commented that the 'puzzle continues to intrigue', it was at that time little explored, and there was little reference in the British anthropological literature to actual or imputed psychological processes. In the Durkheimian tradition, ritual was, in the main, accepted as an intense socialising experience and left at that. Yet it was not totally uncharted territory. From the literature that has developed since then (I exclude psychoanalysis as beyond my present purposes), it is evident that the commentary can be seen largely as elaborations on the theories advanced by Malinowski (1945) and Radcliffe-Brown (1952) on the relationship between anxiety and ritual.

In simplest terms ritual, for Malinowski, serves as a means of allaying the anxieties evoked by the uncertainty of life, whilst for Radcliffe-Brown it acts to induce anxiety as a means of reinforcing social values (*cf.* Homans 1941). For Malinowski, the function of ritual was seen from the point of view of the individual for whom it created necessary confidence; for Radcliffe-Brown, its function was seen from the point of view of society, and interpreted as providing an intense socialising experience. The Malinowskian version, in the form of a cathartic model of the ritual process, has been the more widely used.

Indeed Scheff (1977) defines ritual in just such terms, and it is central to the work of Turner (1967) and Girard (1977) also. Mentioned by Aristotle, and given further dimensions in the work of Freud, the theory of catharsis has many variants. Without going into the complexities, the common strands, as applied to ritual, are firstly, a prior situation of tension or conflict and secondly, the enactment or representation of this in the ritual with a consequent purging of emotional affect for the participants. This model was used by Gluckman (1963) to give force to his 'rituals of rebellion' thesis, and it appears in several different guises in the work of Turner (1967). But clearly, not all ritual, or violence in ritual, involves catharsis – a position I intend to illustrate by comparing a situation where it does, with Gisu circumcision, where I argue it does not.

From the point of view of a comparison with the Gisu, an interesting example is provided by the studies of the Ilongot headhunters of the Philippines by Michelle and Renato Rosaldo. The Ilongot structure their perceptions of the capacities of manhood in terms of *liget* (energy/anger/passion) – a concept which, on the face of it, has evident similarities with the Gisu *lirima*. Among the Ilongot, however, *liget* is counterpoised to *beya*, 'knowledge', which ideally should inform and govern the raw vitality of *liget*. *Liget* is characteristic of youth and it is the passion behind, and also realised and transcended in, the 'tossing of heads' – the triumphant end of a successful head-hunting raid. Then the individual simultaneously proves himself to be the equal of other men in the power of his 'anger', and 'casts' this anger off, lightening his 'heavy heart'. M. Rosaldo writes, 'the gay victors ... purged of violence ... will seek out flowery reeds to wear like feathers signifying lightness' (1980: 55). R. Rosaldo elaborates:

> To take a head is, in Ilongot terms, not to capture a trophy, but to 'throw away' a body part, which by a principle of sympathetic magic represents the cathartic throwing away of certain burdens of life – the grudge an insult has created, or the grief over a death in the family, or the increasing 'weight' of remaining a novice when one's peers have left that status.
>
> (1980: 140)

To summarise, head-hunting is presented as primarily a cathartic act, celebrated in songs as the source of individual and communal strength and joy.

Gisu circumcision lacks these kinds of connotations. Among the Ilongot the young, by definition, have *liget*, and it is *liget* which is seen to inspire the desire to head-hunt. But among the Gisu *lirima* is induced in the course of the ritual, and any catharsis appears as an unstressed by-product. Thus there is obvious relief after the operation; the boy is described as pure and clean, and in a state of passivity his *lirima* is dissipated and inert. For the relatives and spectators, also whipped into a state of intense excitement, the aftermath of the operation is a time for quiet sociability (of drinking beer together in the compound) – though there is also the further drama of the arrival of the father's age mates to demand their customary dues of gifts, as well as continuing anxiety over the boy's health. Relief, however, is not catharsis, and to look at the Gisu ritual in terms of cathartic release would be distorting. The emphasis in Gisu circumcision is not on the release or transcendence of *lirima*, but upon its creation. The power is proved, not purged or transformed into something else.

We turn now to the alternative model, where ritual is seen to achieve its effects through the creation of anxiety. A good example is Spencer's use of 'anxiety intensification' ideas to account for the psychological effects of initiation among the Kenyan Samburu. He suggests:

> That at a time when social relationships are undergoing change, the uncertainties of the occasion which Malinowski saw as a cause for anxiety, and the beliefs and ritual prescriptions which Radcliffe-Brown saw as an additional cause for anxiety, may serve to induce a mental state in the participants which implements these changes. ... They increase the suggestibility of the participants so that they come to accept the change.
>
> (Spencer, 1965; quoted in Spencer, 1970: 144–46)

Spencer draws on Sargant's *Battle for the Mind* (1957) to give an additional psycho-physiological account of the process. Sargant's explication is by reference to Pavlov's experiments on the conditioning of dogs, where it was found that when animals are subjected to extreme stress habitual behaviour patterns are disrupted, and in such 'transmarginal' states new behaviour patterns can be induced and remain stable after recovery. From this, Sargant argues that the induction of extreme anxiety, fatigue and forms of physical debilitation are major techniques for political and religious conversion.

A similar 'brainwashing' effect, Spencer maintains, can be adduced in Samburu circumcision, with the rites impressing upon initiates the ideas of honour and the authority of elders. The rites can be seen to prepare the initiates for a prolonged period – ten or more years – of glamorous but deprived *moranhood* (warriorhood), effectively expelled from the society with wealth and wives being concentrated in the hands of the elders.

There are obvious elements of trauma in Gisu circumcision, and it might well be plausible to adduce this in order to explain the great emotional reaction that adult Gisu men display throughout their lives to the event, as well as (possibly) why the only formal 'teaching' of the boy that occurs takes place so soon after the operation – the circumciser returning during the night, or, at the latest, early on the morning after circumcision. This last episode is brief but important. The boy is first ritually washed and then handed, one by one, the main accoutrements of adult life. Nevertheless, the values associated with Gisu circumcision, and the atmosphere surrounding it, are sufficiently different from that of the Samburu to make it necessary to look elsewhere for a model of its psychic effectiveness.

Let me expand this difference. One matter of interest is that while Spencer records little information on the preparation of Samburu boys for the ordeal, he notes, 'During the twenty-four hours before the first circumcisions they were generally subdued, a number of them shivered, at least one of them developed a facial twitch and another a fixed frown' (1965: 254). And, if the initiates were anxious, a situation of near panic seems to have been characteristic of the onlookers as doubts grew as to whether the boys would stand courageously. Spencer writes that some of the existing *moran* broke down and shook insensibly, while there was the active threat of an affray after one *moran* attempted to strike an initiate who had the temerity to sing of his courage (ibid.: 105).[3] And throughout, he emphasises the relatively passive role of the initiates: the ceremony 'in every detail and at every stage ... was under the control of the elders ... The initiates had to do at each stage what they were told. From beginning to end they seemed thoroughly bewildered' (ibid.: 255).

The contrasting themes of Gisu circumcision are: first, that the boy is going to be made formally equal to his seniors; second, that throughout the ceremony it is he, and not the elders, who is presented as being in control of the situation; lastly, and most importantly for this discussion, that the boy ought to have overcome his anxiety by the time he enters the circumcision enclosure. To this end, the greatest emphasis is on various preparatory rituals, which normally go on for several weeks prior to the operation. The expectation that the boy should betray no sign of fear involves considerably more than simply not flinching at the end. Ideally, he should be completely relaxed. 'Go, as if it were a mere song', I have heard it said. The conscious psychological frame, as well as the structural situation, is thus different. This suggests that if we are looking for parallels in the area of behaviourist psychology then we should look not at ideas relating to 'brainwashing', but to the possibly more straightforward idea of 'battleproofing'.

Battleproofing consists of enacting situations of danger, so allowing the person to become accustomed to, and inured against, fear. Peter Watson (1980) writes that military training is most effective when it gives experience of situations of stress of a kind that allow the men to develop confidence in their ability to face danger. Battleproofing, the process of desensitising the person to danger, is a concept used by military psychologists and it appears to be equally a part of the pragmatic psychology used by the army. An example, in this case reported in a regional English paper, is the brief account of abseiling exercises by sixteen-year-old army recruits. The major in charge explained that the exercises were very good for building up a young soldier's character, 'They've got to overcome their fear and it's very important for a soldier to know that he can conquer his fear'. These exercises started with 100-foot drops and ended with the 'death slide', a drop over a precipice into a river, hitting it at a speed of thirty miles per hour. This, I suggest, is the kind of common-sense vision which the Gisu would immediately comprehend.

The Gisu ritual can be seen to have the same clear-cut aims and techniques; these are particularly apparent in the preparatory rituals, and can be briefly summarised. Firstly, the emphasis is put on the boy being 'strong' enough (kamani). This 'strength' implies both physical strength and what we would call strength of purpose. It is evidenced in the vigour with which the boy dances and in the jumps which effectively rehearse the final jump he will make to face the circumcisers. Second, the boy is subjected to repeated exhortations by elders and bystanders. They tell him of the ordeal he faces, and how he must stand it. There is never at any stage anything secret about the ordeal; no mystery. Further, he is continually asked if he is sure he can go through with it and urged to withdraw if he has any doubt. He may withdraw, without shame, at any time up to actually entering the circumcision enclosure for the operation. On the ritual level, his determination is tested by a series of smearing rites which are explicitly interpreted as mortifications – as unpleasant and abhorrent – and done to 'anger' him, to incite his lirima and spur him on. Additionally, he is encouraged to prepare himself in other ways, for example by pinching his foreskin to give himself some idea of the pain, and so on.

Culture and the ambiguity of violence

Let me move towards a conclusion. In the previous section I indicated very briefly three different ways in which violence has been seen
to have psychological effects in rituals involving ordeals. The examples
used have been selective and were chosen to illustrate these processes
and provide easy points of comparison with the Gisu material. I have
also been concerned to simplify, and it is not suggested that these
rituals necessarily utilise only one such mode or that those outlined
exhaust the possibilities. Clearly, at one level, it is a matter of
emphasis; complex rituals may elicit a wide range of responses in the
participants, just as concentration on different phases of the ritual may
yield very different interpretations. Nevertheless, such rituals are
plainly not all the same type of event, and three main psychological
processes can, I suggest, be usefully distinguished:

1   catharsis: in which negative emotions are turned into positive
    ones;
2   trauma: where the ordeal is seen to have a chastening or even a
    destabilising effect on the individual, and is an aspect of repressive
    socialisation;
3   battleproofing (or disinhibition, as the psychologists term it):
    which involves the use of violence to harden and prepare the indi-
    vidual for violence.

It may be noted that with both catharsis and trauma, violence could be
a technique used in ritual, a means of creating or maintaining values
which in themselves have little or no intrinsic connection with
violence in the non-ritual context – values such as lightening 'heavy
hearts', honour, the authority of elders, and so on. However, this is not
to deny that the ritual would tend to generate an association and,
among both the Ilongot and Samburu where there are clear continu-
ities between the violence in ritual and in secular life, it is difficult to
establish any sharp distinction. Nevertheless, I would argue that
battleproofing is somewhat different, since here the means are more
directly adapted to the ends. Violence is used to breed violence in a
more obvious way. It is also, perhaps because of this obviousness, the
least interesting as a psychological process. However, what we appear
to have in Gisu circumcision is a particularly clear example of it.

Yet, if Gisu circumcision as an ordeal seems simple at this level,
then the question of both the effects and stability of such experiences
on the personality structure looms large. What exactly is the effect of

the experience on the boys? In this respect, I suppose one would like to know whether ordeals of this kind do have a long-lasting effect, not only in inuring the individual against pain, fear and violence, but possibly predisposing the individual, or susceptible individuals, to violence thereafter. If the Gisu ritual operates in an analogous way to military training, encouraging men to react in specific ways to certain forms of stress, does it create, in turn, a greater readiness to use violence and to react aggressively at a later time? Is there some form of trigger effect?

As I indicated earlier, there are reasons for this being an interesting line of inquiry in the Gisu case, even if it is outside the scope of this chapter. I assume that, in most cultural situations, the psychological or psycho-physiological arousal induced is difficult to separate from more general value orientations; that is, the cognitive frame would be compatible with and validate violent responses towards certain stimuli.[4] Military training in Western countries is a case in point. But this is not so unproblematic for the Gisu for, as I have said, although *lirima* has positive value and is regarded as essential for standing the ordeal bravely it is also seen to create 'dangerous' men. Indeed, the Gisu see their life as plagued by men of violence whose *lirima* may bubble up at the slightest provocation and where it is a constant facet of the personality. Further, this kind of aggressive response is *not* culturally condoned (far from it), and may indeed lead to the offenders being killed.

If one follows this line of thinking then one is faced with a kind of paradox. Circumcision is of central cultural significance: it is tradition in its most valued sense, not only signifying but ensuring the continuity of the people and their distinctive ancestry and heritage. That Gisu boys still desire circumcision is a sign that the ancestors are still a force active in Gisu life and, by the same token, the Gisu believe that if they forswore the custom then they would all die out. Given the strength of such sentiments, it seems unthinkable to suppose that it could disappear. But, from another point of view, it is an anachronism. It seems to be fairly widely accepted that ordeals of this kind are linked to warfare. They are a form of training for the bravery and stoicism of the warrior. Elsewhere in East Africa this association holds, and the evidence is well summarised by Ocaya-Lakidi. The ideal tribal virtue of manly excellence, he writes, was strongly connected to warfare and 'led the Eastern African societies to place undue emphasis on masculinity and manliness, the one to be tested sexually and the other in hot combat' (1979: 152). Ultimately, however, the two tests were one, and taking the Kikuyu as an example he elaborates, 'the lengthy initiation rites gave ample opportunity for gauging a man's masculinity, while the supreme pain of circumcision tested his manliness and suitability for warriorhood. That is why becoming a man meant access to physical sex and to warriorhood at the same time' (ibid.:152).

In a large number of East African societies, male gender identity linked to circumcision has therefore a strong military accent, yet for the majority of these societies the warfare and raiding patterns in which this developed are no longer relevant. Some seventy years after pacification this is certainly the case for the Gisu, just as it is for the Kikuyu and for the Samburu discussed earlier. In the Gisu case all that remains of the association is the idea that the fortitude required of the circumcision candidate is akin to the courage of the warrior. An analogy is drawn: a boy must have faith in his powers and strength in the same way that the warrior has faith in his. But I never heard it suggested that the ritual either would or should make him a good fighter. Indeed, such is definitely *not* the aim. Significantly, of the objects of adult life handed to him in the cleansing rite after the operation, a spear is not included. It is perhaps notable by its absence: the boy receives food, fire, a panga, a hoe and a drinking tube; he is told to use these objects properly, in a socially productive way and not for violence and disruption. Thus the circumciser, as he hands the boy a piece of smouldering firewood, says:

> Kindle this piece of firewood and as you kindle it I say, 'Do not go and burn down the houses of your neighbours. I have made you kindle it so that your wife can cook for you and you can heat water and make tea for yourself' ...
> I give you this panga and say, 'Build a house, do not just roam around. I have given you this panga so that you can fell trees and build a house, cut down bananas and banana stems to plant so that you will have your own food. Let me give you this knife so that you can do this work, let me not give it so that you go and attack your neighbours. Nor have I given it to you so you can go and steal the cows of your neighbours and then slaughter them' ...
> I give you this drinking tube to hold and say, 'Drink beer and brew it. Do not get drunk and quarrelsome so that you are always fighting with your friends ...'

I include this long extract from one such speech which I recorded in order to demonstrate the extent to which the dangers of misuse are dramatically reiterated. That the individual is admonished in this way by moral injunctions highlights the fact that there are seen to be few other checks on violence. Its use is seen to be a matter of personal disposition: the good man controls his anger, the bad man does not.

At this point one is tempted to compare the Gisu concept of manhood with others in East Africa. As indicated above, many equally extol martial virtues, but in the modern era not all of these have feared male violence in the same way. The Kikuyu are a case in point and, as a related Bantu-speaking people, their concepts bear direct comparison with those of the Gisu. For the Kikuyu the cardinal virtues of the warrior combine fierceness with restraint. *Urume*, the quality par excellence of the warrior (*injamba*), has evident affinity with the Gisu *lirima*, implying bravery, determination in the face of adversity and violent forceful action.[5] Men may shake with *urume*, a physical manifestation which is widely recognised among both the Bantu and para-Nilotic peoples of Kenya as a sign of courage and, more especially, readiness for battle. At the same time, the Kikuyu warrior was expected to display the virtues of identification and loyalty to his age set, and obedience and submission to the authority of seniors. Disciplined self-control thus emerges as a major theme in Kikuyu life, with a man expected to exercise restraint both in his use of violence and, indeed, in sex (Kenyatta, 1938). In this gerontocratic social order, warriorhood was only part of a process of individual self-development, orchestrated by age-group status; circumcision marked only the beginning of the achievement of the full potentialities of manhood. In this respect, and in their military traditions, the Kikuyu appear similar to the Samburu discussed earlier. Speaking of the Meru, closely-related to the Kikuyu, Fadiman notes that the process of 'hardening' for a Meru warrior involved a whole series of ordeals and beatings, where a true warrior 'was expected to show neither weakness in the face of pain, nor resistance to those who applied it' (Fadiman, 1982: 49). Indeed, he writes that most of the pain a warrior was expected to bear was inflicted by members of his own community. As with the Kikuyu, the warrior was part of a disciplined fighting force which came under the direction of elders.

In so far as these historically forged attitudes persist we may perhaps find clues to the different perceptions of the capacity of men for violence. From the previous discussion what emerges as a significant shaper of attitudes is age-set organisation, traditionally absent in Bugisu. Among the Gisu named age sets were formed to include boys circumcised at the same time, generally every two years; such men were held to have special bonds with each other, a comradeship developed in the months of curing and presumably tested in the subsequent fighting. But such sets did not form standing corps of warriors, nor did they collectively progress through a series of set ranks based on age status. Thus, while self-discipline is a valued quality, it is not stressed to any great degree and receives little institutional support. Rather than to age status and to the submission to the group and its leaders, the greater weight is given to the essential equality of all men, won on a kind of once-and-for-all basis through the ordeal of circumcision.

If rites of passage are regarded not only as transition markers but also as transformational experiences, then the possible effects on individual consciousness, and indeed on character structure, loom large. It is then no longer sufficient to see initiation rituals simply as formal markers of status or as part of the regulatory mechanism whereby social classifications are maintained and social life made predictable and orderly. As Herdt comments, 'a narrow sociological paradigm no longer seems adequate' (Herdt, 1982:480). Indeed, when the focus shifts to the individual then what has been revealed is the often paradoxical nature of the rituals, sometimes in conflict with secular values and deeply disturbing to the participants. The ethnography coming from New Guinea (ibid.) vividly makes this point, with the male cults there designed to create fierce warriors based on a cruelty which is at variance with other values of community and domestic life, and creating their own poignant moral dilemmas. With the cessation of warfare in recent years some of these peoples have gladly abandoned their cults or the more repugnant aspects of them. The Gisu rites do not involve cruelty in the same way. The Gisu dilemma is perhaps most easily seen as a variant on the problem of what to do with the warriors when there is no war to fight. If they have adapted to the extent of expunging the more obviously bellicose connotations from their rites, these rituals still leave them defined as a nation of violent men if not as a nation of warriors.

4

EVERY MAN A HERO
Oedipal themes in Gisu circumcision

How should an anthropologist use psychoanalysis? What can it add to our accounts? My starting position here is that it provides a hermeneutic which invites us to reinterrogate our data in order to both challenge and augment the interpretations already made on the basis of more standard forms of exegesis. In the Durkheimian tradition within which I have broadly worked, cultural values are taken to be relatively straightforwardly depicted in cultural symbolism. By contrast, psychoanalysis tells us that the symbolic process is complex, bedevilled by the forces of repression, whereby the manifest becomes a mask or, at best, a distorting mirror to psychic reality. If custom may be taken as symbolic in the psychoanalytic sense, speaking to unconscious fantasy and process, then it has the capacity to turn our accepted interpretive canons upside down. In so doing, it does not, of course, invalidate the cultural interpretation. Devereux's postulate of 'complementarity' is essential here, though it is today less easy to see, as he did, that the coming together of the two perspectives will give a determinate understanding in either.[1]

For many anthropologists the first fieldwork is the most formative experience of our lives and sets the agenda for much of what we do later. For me, it established a long-lasting source of intrigue with the topic of male circumcision. For the Gisu of Uganda, circumcision presents itself as a particularly severe ordeal which boys are required to undergo roughly between the ages of seventeen and twenty-five in order to validate their claims to manhood. In Chapter Two, I have explored it from the point of view of what I called their 'vernacular psychology', how the Gisu see it as actually creating men, an identity forged in the ritual process. In Chapter Three, I have tried to trace out the concordances of this process with its transformational potential and western psychological theories, drawn largely from behaviourist psychology. In neither did I consider psychoanalysis. This is the challenge which I now take up and it is one which allows me to probe new areas, going beneath the overt level of culturally interpreted symbolism to look at how sexuality is encoded in the ritual. The challenge is, however, not without difficulties.

The first problem is epistemological. Anthropological commentary on psychoanalysis has frequently criticised it for its unprovable assumptions and analysis. For example, Leach castigates psychoanalysis for its 'atrocious methods of hit or miss intuition' (1958: 149). This critique has always seemed inappropriate, as is the case when the pot calls the kettle black. As Cohen writes 'psychoanalysis has at least as much claim to be considered a body of "scientific" ideas as do most others that are used by anthropologists in the study of symbolism' (1980: 48). Further, just as anthropology has reoriented its quest away from positivistic and natural science models of inquiry and towards more hermeneutic forms of understanding, so, too, a similar move has been argued for psychoanalysis. For Ricoeur (1979), Freud's true discovery lies in the realm of meaning, in the hermeneutics of suspicion, and thus in unravelling the deceptions of consciousness. The problems of validation of an interpretation are perhaps here no different from those that the anthropologist normally has to deal with; the unconscious dynamic must be shown to have some external correlative, either in the experience of the individual or in cultural practice. Nevertheless, whether in meaning or mechanism, the psychoanalytical model here frequently has an alternative mode of validation – which anthropology lacks – in its therapeutic claims. Thus, fantasy, symbol and ritual are deemed to have an observable effect on the emotional adjustment of individuals.

The second problem is to try to make sense of the claims made and to choose between rival readings of the 'theory'. Probably, the dominant line of argument relating to the practice of circumcision in the anthropological literature has its roots in Freud and the dynamics involved in the 'family romance', as he called it.[2] In the most general terms, circumcision has been seen as a response to ineffectual repression of the Oedipal conflict in infancy. In adolescence, after the latency period, this has been seen to lead to a renewal of desire for the mother accompanied by hostile rivalry with the father. Further cultural buttresses are then seen as being required in order to solve the problems of psychic adjustment for individuals in these cultures, for example, by reinvoking castration anxiety through the practice of circumcision accompanied by taboos on sexual contact with senior women, taboos which have been seen as phobic responses to incest (see Reik (1931) and after him Stephens and D'Andrade (1962)). The ritual then is seen to involve some kind of mimesis of the repressed conflicts encountered in childhood and the therapeutic dynamic is that of cathartic abreaction, serving to reconcile the son to his father's authority, to the cultural values which he represents and, most significantly, to the incest taboo.

In this context, Gisu circumcision presents itself initially as a striking negative example. It is an act which grants full adult status to a man and, in so doing, emancipates him from his father's authority. Further, there is no repression of antagonism. Indeed, circumcision marks the assumption of the most intense competition between father and son over the question of inheritance and this competition frequently results in violence. If we take manifest behaviour then, we cannot conclude the circumcision in this case effects the kind of reconciliation between father and son, a decrease in their rivalry, that we might expect.

How then should we read the theory? Do we conclude that the Oedipal conflict is either not universal or that resolution of it is not necessary? One problem here is that it is often not clear what 'resolution' means when anthropologists – or, indeed, psychoanalysts – invoke the concept. Is it, for example, a true resolution or does it involve further repression, with perhaps a new *modus vivendi*, but one equally liable to intra-psychic conflict? Further, if the process is largely unconscious, how are we to make the inferences we need for an evaluation? Unlike the psychoanalyst, the anthropologist has no transference material by which to validate his or her hypotheses. In part – but only in part – these problems arise from the type of causal developmental theory being used here, a theory which still sees culture as a 'psychic defense system', as Roheim (1934) put it, and which has not taken on the messages from more recent neo-Freudian work with its less deterministic framework. Psychoanalysis, like anthropology, has moved on and it is perhaps time to look at material such as initiation rites not so much as – or perhaps, not only as – in the business of 'therapy' but as conveying messages about the way attachment to and detachment from the mother and resentment of the father may be handled in the particular cultural setting. If we take this as a starting point, it is apparent that the messages could be at variance with each other and may recapitulate conflicts without necessarily solving them. Ricoeur (1979; 1981) sees in Freud's genius not the pairing of symbol with a determinant meaning but the idea that the operations of fantasy betray no automatic laws, just as psychoanalysts find that individuals deal differently with reality and the defensive mechanisms they develop are labial and not fixed.

The choice in the interpretation of ritual then could be phrased as a choice between a developmental version which gives primacy to the formative experiences of childhood and sees ritual as emerging to solve these or a cultural account which gives priority to the ordering of symbolic meaning. In so far as this latter approach shifts the emphasis from the individual to culture it shifts the interpretation from a determinate psycho-dynamic developmental schema to a more variable one. Thus, the unconscious is seen as a resource which might be used to add emotive power to the ritual process and its dominant symbols, but without the implications of necessity. Among Africanists, it is well represented in the work of Fortes and Turner, both of whom managed to weld psychoanalytic insights into an otherwise Durkheimian perspective. For Durkheim, the key problem in social life was commitment and the role of religion was to galvanise both consciousness and conscience, impressing upon the individual the authority of culture and the supremacy of society. Fortes and Turner [3] both speculate upon how religion utilises the powers of the unconscious to this end, 'domesticating' conflicts, both intra-psychic and inter-personal. Further, Turner (1967) argues that, through the process of condensation, ritual symbols effect a synthesis of referents, drawing upon both emotionally charged physio-psychological processes and normative values. If this seems to give too much primacy to the social, with the idea that the resources of the *libido* are utilised for the purposes of social control, it nevertheless allows for a way of integrating the two perspectives, by emphasising not only the element of social control but also that of individual growth.

Themes in Gisu circumcision

If psychoanalytic understandings are to be used to inform cultural analysis, it is necessary first to outline briefly the dominant themes in Gisu circumcision and its emotional power.

The Gisu live at one end of a broad circumcising belt which runs down from Mount Elgon south and east through Kenya to Tanzania. Everywhere in this area, it would be fair to say, circumcision is strongly linked both to male gender identity and ethnicity. Nowhere is this clearer than in Bugisu. The rituals of *imbalu* are held every two years during the month of August and the boys are required to stand upright for the operation betraying no signs of fear, pain or reluctance. As an ordeal, it thus has a critical personal dimension, an individual proof of masculinity, demonstrated in the courtyard of the boy's father or other senior relative and witnessed by an assembled throng of kin and neighbours.

It is the ordeal which every young boy knows one day he must face and for which he has prepared himself by joining the circumcision parties for many years before he is finally ready to face the knife himself (to 'fall' or 'enter into' *imbalu*). When the time comes and he announces his decision, he is repeatedly told that he only has one chance – 'there is only one knife' – and that he should withdraw if he has any doubts rather than risk failure. Failure threatens on many counts. Most evidently in the display of cowardice or fear, which in extreme cases pollutes the circumcision knife and the compound of his father. But the whole of his adult life is also seen as dependent on *imbalu*. Much then is deemed at stake, but the emotional power of *imbalu* reaches far beyond this.

Undoubtedly, it is the most emotionally-charged occasion for all Gisu men and, indeed, for the whole community, for whom its drama is re-enacted every two years. During the circumcision periods the whole of the countryside rings to the sound of the boys' bells and circumcision songs, and people are whipped up into states of intense excitement as they champion the candidates and urge them to bear it bravely. Dressed in the flamboyant regalia, the boys glory in the glamour of their position at the centre of everyone's attention and concern. Importantly, it is they who are seen as leading the country forward; it is their decision, their volition, their actions which mobilise their kin and their friends behind them. Further, in proving their manhood, they are in effect proving the identity of all Gisu as men and validating the power of the tradition which unites them all. 'Caught' by the ancestral power of circumcision, the boys, in effect, personify the power of the ancestors and the continuity of tradition.

Gisu circumcision is thus presented as a heroic act. Performed at a relatively late age when the boy is already physiologically and sexually mature, the rite can also explicitly be seen as a test of whether he is also, in Gisu terms, 'psychologically' a man, capable of demonstrating the force of character necessary to see through the ritual to completion. The key Gisu concept here is *lirima*, which in the present context can be glossed as 'anger'. The diacritical sign of *lirima* is however in the intensity of the emotion experienced. Thus it is spoken of as 'catching' a man or 'bubbling-up' in him. While in this state of possession, *lirima* is seen to dictate all a man's attitudes and actions; it gives force to motivation and impels to action. In normal life *lirima* is linked to all the negative emotions, to jealousy, hatred, resentment and shame, and is seen as responsible for all the trouble in the community. It is only in circumcision that it is given a positive value. It *must* bubble-up in the initiate so that all his actions are dominated by the over-riding desire to see the ritual through to completion. If a man can be in the grip of *lirima* he can use it to steel himself too.

The intensity of *lirima*, its power and its 'bitterness' make this above all a manly attribute and women and boys are held not to experience it. They are held subject only to the lesser form of arousal of *libuba*. Circumcision thus becomes the first occasion on which a boy is required to display *lirima* and, as I have recounted elsewhere, this capacity then becomes as much a part of his manhood as the circumcision cuts themselves. Indeed, most the symbolism of the preparatory ritual can be explicated in terms of the induction of *lirima*.

The linking of circumcision with the creation of *lirima* in the individual is central to the purposes of the rite. Having faced 'death' he is deemed free from the fear of it and capable of taking full responsibility for himself among other self-determining Gisu men. Indeed, circumcision is the first act of self-determination of a Gisu youth, transforming him from a mere boy, an appendage of his father, to a man, with a status equivalent to his father. It is thus, above all, a rite of emancipation from parental authority and this has important political and economic correlates. After circumcision, a man is expected to marry and set up as an independent householder, responsible for providing for himself and for his own dependants. He no longer is reliant on his natal family for food, or even ritual protection, for he now becomes responsible for protecting his own family and may make sacrifices to the ancestors on his own behalf.

Oedipal accounts: father and son

Given this conscious frame for the interpretation of *imbalu*, it is difficult to tie it to the orthodox Freudian account of the significance of circumcision. Certainly, circumcision makes a son like his father; it clearly defines gender identity for the boy, removing him finally from the house of his mother and giving him the right to a wife and a house of his own. But arguments based on the classic account give a particular causal reading of this process which hinges on the recognition of the father's authority. It is fear of the father which motivates repression and the transference of desire and it is only in this context that circumcision has symbolic value as 'castration'. It makes circumcision an act of submission to the father and simultaneously to what he represents, the legitimate, if onerous, authority of culture, represented in the incest taboo.

The whole tenor of the ritual argues against this. The rite is an act of emancipation and, insofar as one sees it as giving a very forceful stamp to male gender identity and the equivalence of all men, it is difficult to read it as an assertion of parental power.[4] Further, its themes offer a vivid contrast with many other initiation rituals. For example, Gisu boys are not passive initiates, dragged from the security of their homes to face unknown and terrifying ordeals in segregated ritual sites under the supervision of male elders. On the contrary, the ordeal is conceived of as an act of individual volition, with the boy freely choosing his year and thus making manifest the powers and capabilities of his ancestry. Indeed, the ritual exalts the act of individual choice and, in so doing, makes the son and not the father the vector of ancestral continuity. The locus begins and ends with the initiate himself, with the emphasis being upon the particular test of valour which it entails, a valour to which the Gisu give a particular interpretation and psychological meaning.

One way of saving circumcision for an Oedipal reading, however, would be to interpret it as a cultural fantasy serving to disguise the hidden reality of power in order to make it more palatable. But, to be plausible there must be tangible correlates in social arrangements which could be seen as motivating such a fantasy of weak paternal power. But, in Bugisu, parental authority is in reality weak and is accompanied by intense inter-generational conflict which frequently erupts into violence. Parricide is a real threat in Bugisu and so is filicide (La Fontaine, 1967; Heald, 1998). Nor can the operation be deemed to have therapeutic value as, for example, argued by Ottenberg for the Nigerian Afikpo, who saw it as 'an attempt to resolve psychological conflict between father and son, which serves to minimise (but not eliminate) frictions arising out of economic and political issues' (1988: 349). This it signally fails to do among the Gisu for the attribution of violent power to both father and son in effect licenses the use of violence, which becomes a real possibility only after circumcision.

The problems at one level are all structural. After circumcision a father is obliged to provide for his son, that is, to begin to dismember his estate, allocating cattle for bridewealth to allow his son to marry and a parcel of land for him to farm and thus to feed himself and his wife. This obligation is deemed absolute but is, in practice, often difficult to enforce. In the present situation of chronic land shortage, many men have insufficient land and run a serious risk of impoverishment by acceding to their sons' demands. Further, since every man is deemed an equal and in total control of his own affairs, such a distribution is in practice solely at the discretion of the father and no-one has the right to intervene. Father and son are thus engaged in an essentially private dispute; one in which the son's rights are deemed absolute but can only be enforced by the son's own efforts at persuasion which, in the context, also include force.

The fact of circumcision then operates not to underplay competitive rivalry in the father and son relationship but to highlight it. Indeed, for both fathers and sons it creates a situation of double-bind. It establishes the son as an 'equal' but the essential economic resources he needs to establish himself as a full adult, that is, autonomous and self-sufficient, remain still with the father. Indeed, after a relatively free adolescence, circumcision brings to the fore this element of a boy's dependence. However, the way in which it does so serves not to ensure a son's subservience but to intensify the competitive element in their relationship by introducing the possibility of aggression. *Lirima* is deemed necessary for a man to defend his own interests against other men; the direct resort to physical force by the young or to witchcraft by the old is seen to follow from this. This is as likely in the father and son relationship as any other. Indeed, the nature of the competition between them makes it an added threat.

The ambivalence between father and son, seen as the core of the Oedipal complex by Freud, is thus not overcome by circumcision in any simple way. However, it may be seen to dramatically define the terms of the conflict, with the twin imperatives of Oedipus complex – 'be like the father' (i.e., be a man like him) and 'don't be like the father' (i.e., don't take what is his, the mother) – reformulated in the contrast between aggression and sexuality. If the imperative to be 'like the father' is defined in terms of anger and autonomy – in effect, licensing competition in this area – the imperative to be 'not like the father' is defined with respect to sexual prerogatives, outlawing competition in this particular sphere.

The generational divide with respect to sexuality and marriage in Bugisu is absolute. Women of the adjacent generation are totally prohibited and this includes both kinswomen and in-marrying affines. This rule clearly separates the sexual interests of fathers and sons.[5] At its simplest, women are divided into two major categories: those of the adjacent generation, whether kinswomen or affines, who are totally prohibited, and those of one's own generation with whom one has a legitimate sexual interest. The generational patterning of sexual rights tends to override other distinctions in terms of consanguinity and sisters are, to this extent, substitute wives. This is clearly marked in the circumcision rituals.

Sisters – younger real sisters and also those of the kindred – accompany the boy during the last three days leading up to circumcision and are ritually smeared with millet yeast together with the boy. Later, again with the initiate, they are cleansed by the circumciser after the operation and instructed on their role as future wives. At the time of first smearing, they are addressed as his 'wives' and this is usually explained in terms of the right a boy has to use some of their bridewealth in order to marry a wife of his own. While this applies most clearly to the boy's own younger sisters, it also applies by extension to more distant female kin since it is considered that marriages are contracted on behalf of the generation as a whole. These men may inherit each other's wives and compensation for adultery cannot be exacted. No such privileges are accorded between the generations. Thus, while all other forms of property are transmitted vertically, from seniors to juniors, sexual prerogatives are restricted to the generations, clearly demarcating the legitimate zones of interest for fathers and sons.

Fathers and sons may thus not compete sexually.[6] Indeed, the total opposition of the roles of mother and wife is a clear motif in Gisu life, and this finds expression in the way intimate relationships between the sexes are patterned. Women may only stand in one relationship to a man, either as a 'mother' or as a 'wife' and this is realised in particular taboos which restrict the breast to infants. Thus a man should not touch his wife's breasts and nor should she touch his genitalia for it is considered that that is a maternal role, for it is the mother who cleanses a man when he is young. Indeed, even when adult, if a man is ill and incontinent, it must be a woman related to him as a 'mother' who undertakes his physical care. Thus the Gisu are offered two possible but mutually incompatible models of conduct towards the opposite sex, that which might be called conjugal sexuality and the other, generative consanguinity.

If the transformation of desire from 'mothers' to 'sisters' is thus depicted in the ritual, this raises the question of how this effect might be achieved on a psychodynamic level. The mere picturing of the legitimate relationships, won through circumcision, though it forcefully expresses cultural propriety, raises the problem of how this is made palatable and how the ritual itself might be seen as aiding such a process. With this in mind, I now turn to the way in which sexuality is depicted in the rites.

Sexual symbolism

There are in fact few specifically sexual symbols at circumcision but, nevertheless, it is underwritten by a symbolism of process and powerful metaphors of sexuality and gestation run through it. These hinge on the symbolism of beer and fermentation. The whole ritual process is orchestrated with reference to the making of millet beer. The threshing of the millet for this beer is the first ritual act performed by the initiate and it is taken to signify intent. Later he initiates the last three-day fermentation cycle which leads up to his own circumcision by pouring water on the prepared millet and at the same time he is smeared from head to toe with millet yeast; the same yeast that is added to the brew. I have emphasised in previous chapters how this draws together two processes: the fermentation of beer and the development of *lirima* in the boy. The bubbling volatility of beer and its transformative powers provide a fitting metaphor for the fundamental nature of the change which the boy is deemed to be undergoing and this is directly linked to the growth of his 'anger'. But, beer-making also provides an important model by which the Gisu understand the process of gestation. Thus, pregnancy in women is likened to fermentation, with the 'white blood' of the man and the 'red blood' of the woman described as mixing together to form a child. Beer-making thus exemplifies creative process, whether of fermentation, gestation and or that involved in becoming a man.

In the course of the ritual attention is drawn to the similarity between these processes by a series of shouts. Firstly, as the boy pours the water on the beer, the shout goes up, 'You have spoilt it'. When he himself is circumcised, usually following the first cut, this is marked by the shout, 'They have spoilt you'. Lastly, one other event is marked in this way and that is when a girl is deflowered on her wedding night. Then it is said, 'He has spoilt you'. This constitutes an extended metaphor which can be unpacked in a number of ways.

In the first place, the word 'spoilt' is very definitely polysemic for the Gisu and carries a range of connotations. At one end it clearly designates our normal usage, something which has been subject to change and thus ruined: a useless thing. It is also applied to the spoiling of children through over-indulgence. Of the 'spoiling' at circumcision it may thus be said that the boy has been made useless and will not be able to engage in sexual intercourse or indeed in any normal life until he is finally cured. But, at the other end of the scale, spoiling is seen as necessary precondition for generative potential. Indeed, through the three shouts, explicit attention is being drawn to the parallels between circumcision, defloration and the adding of water to the brew. One idea that clearly links these occasions is the necessity for an original integrity of substance or persons to be destroyed in order for them to later fulfil their purpose. Water must be added to the millet before the yeast can activate fermentation; women must have their hymen ruptured before they can conceive and, likewise, a man should be cut before he can marry.

The spoiling is thus the necessary act for generation and such 'spoiling' is an achievement of culture. Women and men, no more than beer, are 'naturally' fertile: in all cases human agency has to work on the world of nature to release procreative potentiality and this destruction is performed culturally. The making of women is not more natural than the making of men or the making of beer. Or, to put it another way, natural fertility is created culturally, whether in people or in beer. One can also note that yeast, the generative agency in the case of beer, is also created culturally by germinating millet seeds. Again, when it sprouts, the millet is said to be spoilt. In all cases too, this is seen to lead to an increase in violence and aggression; the bubbling of the beer, the potency of a man linked to *lirima*, and the turbulence created in the process of gestation which is held to explain the irritability of women during pregnancy.

At circumcision, the boys first 'spoils' the millet before himself becoming 'spoilt' and both acts carry the implications of sexuality. Indeed, the act of making beer is directly linked to sexuality and circumcision is the first time in which a boy participates in the task. Thereafter, when he marries, he will help his wife with the making of beer and when they do this they must abstain from sexual intercourse for the three days of the final fermentation lest the beer become 'too strong'. Beer-brewing and sexuality are thus seen to positively interact as processes. With this in mind, we can explore further the significance of the boy making it together with his *mother* at circumcision.

Mother and son

Mother and son make the circumcision beer together, with the mother providing the millet and taking over from her son in completing all the tasks necessary for the final fermentation, including adding the yeast to the brew. In this, she may be seen as in actuality initiating the final fermentation after the, in a sense, false simulation of this when the boy pours the water on the millet. With beer-making as a symbol of fertility and *lirima*, this makes the mother largely responsible for her son's courage just as it represents the mother rebirthing him. Indeed, this is clearly one implication. The mother's identification with her son is absolute and, daubing her face also with yeast, she may symbolically be seen as going through a second birth of her son. This emerges clearly during the actual time of the operation when she retires to her house and takes up the attitude she had when giving birth, either standing or squatting, and often clasping the centre pole of her house.

Would it be too far-fetched to read the beer-making as a representation of the libidinal bonds that bound the mother to her son in childhood? I think this might well be a valid interpretation, accompanied, as it is, with the substitution of wife for mother in the smearing ritual. One reading might be that through her identification and 'rebirthing', the mother is symbolically releasing her son from his attachment to her and freeing him for independent adulthood. But, to give strength to this interpretation, we need to examine further the relationship of mother and son and take this back to infancy.

Since Freud, much psychoanalytic theory has come to emphasise the problems of separation and individuation and this has led to a re-evaluation of the mother and child relationship and the effects of early dependence. The relationship of this to the Oedipal complex itself is variously conceived but for many, including such diverse writers as Klein and Lacan, it involves the postulation of a pre-Oedipal situation in the fusion of the child with the mother in infancy. Childhood can be seen to involve a series of transitions as the child seeks to differentiate himself from his symbiotic union with his mother. For Lacan (1977), the first relationship of a child with the mother is associated with what he calls the mirror phase. This constitutes the first step towards the realisation of subjectivity in the recognition which occurs around six months of age in an infant that he is a 'singular' entity. For Lacan, this is, as yet, an incomplete subjectivity which is only fully realised with the assumption of language when the subject takes on 'the dialectic of identification with the other', a stage which Lacan identifies with the Oedipal complex. The 'father' enters here as the destroyer of the mother/child bond, a destruction necessary for the child to realise his own independent identity. The tangible effects of this for a child are maternal rejection and it is this which constitutes, for Lacan, the symbolic castration. As a universal predicament he postulates that the reaction to the loss must be repression. The desire for the mother is repudiated and made unconscious while the desire for the phallus is deferred.

If we are to look for the roots of individuation in early infancy, it is necessary to say more about this in the Gisu context. Unfortunately, I did not collect systematic data on *post-partum* sexual abstinence, age of weaning or mother-infant sleeping arrangements. Nevertheless, my observations lead me to suppose that weaning today is usually achieved around the end of the first year of life and that *post-partum* sexual taboos are often effectively lifted before the age of weaning. Weaning may be undertaken because of a new pregnancy or for fear of over-indulging the child. Thus a reason given for weaning is often that the child is becoming 'spoilt' and this fear gives a particular colouring to the process, with the child being reprimanded for his reliance on the breast. Here, fortunately, there is information of a kind not usually available to the anthropologist on the traumatic significance that weaning may have.

The journey we must all make

In 1989, Wangusa, a Mugisu from southern Bugisu, published a novel, *Upon this Mountain*, which tells the story of three Gisu boys from child-hood to circumcision. One achieves the ordeal successfully, one fails and thereafter adopts the role of a transvestite and lastly, the narrator himself, having witnessed the humiliation of his friend, decides to take the schoolboy's still shameful option of having the operation done in hospital. Because of the insight this book gives, especially on early childhood experiences, I propose to quote it at length and use it as the basis for future discussion. The novel opens with a vivid account of weaning, the first memory of the narrator, Mwambu, which is here reproduced in a slightly abridged form.

> Many, many millet granaries ago, he was mother's child, and she was the child's mother. And they sat in the shade on the verandah of the main house: mother with her legs stretched in front of her, to let the midday meal sink into her bones; and he fast asleep beside mother, with his head in mother's lap. [...]
>
> And he opened his eyes upon his mother: Mother's face, mother's arms, mother's lap. Tendermost mother as before. And he felt the itch inside him to suck at the breast. To clamber into her cosy, eversure lap and suck.
>
> 'Mother mine,' he said, rising and clambering. But as he reached out for the breast, he tripped over her legs and fell against her womb. And then came the rebuff.
>
> 'Pthwoh!' she spat into his face and pushed him away in visible anger. 'You a man!' His face went into a shocked,

wide-mouthed, close-eyed, noiseless contortion ...'You such a grown-up! ...'

Mother-bad-good-bad-good-why?

'...To go harrassing me for my breast as if it was yours! And after you've just eaten so much food!'

And now the noiseless contortion broke into a shrill, loud and long cry of anguished bafflement. [...]

Everything reeled before him. Reeling millet granary. Reeling world. Trembling sky-line through the tear-drops. Mountain falling into the valleys and valleys falling onto the mountain.

[His crying prompted even harsher retaliation and his mother beat him]

But a very powerful voice saved him.

'Who is that beating Mwambu?' His father's voice! From the house. A strong and concerned voice. [...]

And instantly his toddling feet were fleeing from mother's presence to father's voice, through the instinctively remembered door. Before him was an outstretched arm. And now both arms. And then he found himself lifted by strong arms and placed on a strong soft bed. His father held him close to his breast and said:

'And now do not cry any more,
You are a man ...
Do not cry, mother is bad ...
I will beat her for you.'

(Wangusa, 1989: 1–2)

Clearly, the value of this account does not rest on its literal accuracy as to whether weaning is always achieved in this sudden and harsh way. Rather, it gives vivid testimony to the psychic importance of the event; an insight into the effects of maternal rejection and also into the patterning of social relations and their cultural values. Of interest here is that the ambivalent feelings associated with weaning are, in this account, attributed solely to the mother. There is no paternal interdiction. Indeed the male world is presented as the succouring one, the father aligning with his son against the – at that time – inexplicable cruelty of the mother. The novel records how he learnt that his rejection was due to his mother's pregnancy with his younger sister. Further, what is again striking about this account is that the rejection of the breast, immediately qualifies the boy as a 'man', repeated by both the father and his cousin's wife, who offers him the sexual rewards of adult-hood.

> Some days later Mayuba, the newly-married wife of his cousin Kuloba, came into the courtyard and threw him a challenge:
> 'How are you, husband of mine?' she asked. 'I hear that you're no longer sucking mother's breast. You've done a very good thing. And it shows how very wise you are! You've seen that you're now a big man. And that's the truth. And on my part, I am myself now completely ready to be your wife. Tell me, aren't you happy? I'm happy myself ... Come, let's go to our house. Tonight you must share my bed with me. Come at once and let's go to our house ...Come let's go, I say. I am your wife. Your brother has gone on a journey today and I have no husband. You must come and keep his place in the bed warm ...Hey, are you running away? What are you afraid of? Poor me, what a husband ...!'
>
> (Wangusa, 1989: 3)

Reading this account it struck me that circumcision, replaying these same themes, might well draw some of its emotive power from them, and the tangle of emotions which is here presented as unresolved. Can we see in this weaning the symbolic castration that Lacan refers to? The child loses its mother but cannot yet assume the role of an adult and identify with his father or make the immediate transfer from non-genital to genital sexuality. He, in effect, enters a long period characterised by loss, where the mother is no longer 'mine' and clearly has to be shared with the father as well as with his other siblings. The process of autonomous self-development is now marked by a succession of movements away from the mother. From the 'mother mine' of infancy, the son continues to reside in the parental house but with a demoted status, sharing his mother with his father as well as other siblings. At eight or nine years old he makes a further move away when he moves out of the parental home. At this time he either builds himself a boy's house at the edge of his father's compound or goes to live with a friend.

Boys thus differentiate and achieve autonomy in a three-stage move: weaning, extrusion from the parental home and lastly circumcision. The time of his adolescence, when he lives apart from his parents, appears much as an interregnum in his relationship with them. During this time, he is largely freed from direct supervision and parental discipline, always somewhat erratic in Bugisu, is attenuated. Nevertheless, he has yet to gain a full social identity and is still regarded an adjunct to that of his parents. Thus, if ill-luck or illness strike him this is seen as aimed not so much at himself but at his parents. Circumcision dramatically changes this state of affairs; like weaning it marks an abrupt change in his relationship to his parents. It is thus relevant to compare how his relationships with his mother and father are depicted in the ritual, and at how they might relate to the weaning experience.

If we look firstly at the mother's role in the ritual, it is clear that she is presented as expediting her son's assumption of manhood and, in effect, as discussed earlier, 'rebirthing' him. Yet this is a rebirthing where the son himself is seen as the initiator of the process of separation. Circumcision thus effectively reverses the attitudes engendered by weaning as recorded by Wangusa. The mother now is presented in a totally positive light and the separation which marks his final exit from the maternal home is presented as a matter of *his choice*, albeit facilitated by his mother.

There are interesting and important contrasts with the father's role. Again, ideally, the father is presented as nurturant, ensuring his son's safe and successful circumcision by choosing the ritual elder (often himself), and the circumciser and making sure that no ill-will remains in the family which could threaten the boy's welfare. However, he remains on the sidelines, responsible for practical arrangements but not implicated in the actual process whereby his son achieves his manhood. In this, he is rather as the bride's mother in an English wedding and again, like her, he is given no direct role in the ritual itself. Indeed, it is not even important that he be present as long as he has given his permission for it to go ahead, for circumcisions can be performed also at the house of any senior relative, matrilateral as well as patrilineal. But, in any event, the father's role is tinged with ambiguity for the very powers he is entrusted with to ensure his son's well-being are subject to abuse. Thus when a boy fails in the ordeal, fails to show the requisite courage or fails in afterlife and does not manage to maintain a marriage, then directly or indirectly the father may be deemed at fault. No such blame attaches to the mother whose fortitude is always linked in a positive way to that of her son. The same applies also to the sisters who identify strongly with their brothers as they accompany them on the three days leading to circumcision.

One question which must be addressed here is why is the mother idealised? Given the account of weaning, with its horrifying images of alienation and loss of security, a loss which the novel implies is never repaired, why do we not find images of evil female power? We may here refer to the work of Klein who stresses the conflicting attitude of the child to the breast as both the source of libidinal satisfaction and the primary source of frustration. Frustration she held to be inevitable because of the nature of infantile narcissism and omnipotence. The image of the 'bad breast' and bad mother then becomes the 'prototype of all persecuting and frightening objects' (Klein, 1989: 66), a product of the child's aggressive fantasies, which is later carried over to the penis. For Klein, the transfer to genital sexuality is never total and the attitude taken to the breast underwrites the possibility of successful adaptation to mature sexual identity, of a positive attitude to the penis. In Wangusa's account of weaning, the substitution of the penis for the nipple is clearly depicted, as is the ambivalence to the mother. Perhaps, we may also see in the symbolism of the knife which 'eats' the boy's penis at circumcision an indication of oral/sadistic fantasy, a product of the guilt inspired in the child who, through the introjection of threatening parental images, turns his own aggressive fantasies against himself. Circumcision then is not necessarily solely a representation of 'castration' inflicted by fathers but equally, and perhaps more, a representation of the fantasies inspired by maternal rejection.

Whether or not such an interpretation, resting on the intangibility of infantile sexual fantasy, is valid, we can still unite Klein and Lacan with Wangusa and see weaning as the first encounter of the child with the reality principle. Circumcision might then be seen as the test of whether the individual has faced this crisis successfully. The pain of the rejection at weaning is matched by the physical pain born at circumcision and the necessity for the individual to prove he can cope with the hardships and deprivations of life.

To return to the question of why the representation of maternal hostility might be subdued we need again to refer to the structural situation which creates a very real dependence of men upon women. The Gisu inherit through the house-property complex; that is a man has a right only to those fields farmed by his own mother, a prerogative which is especially important in a polygamous household. Mothers are thus crucial intermediaries in a man's struggle to gain his inheritance from his father. Thus the rival claims of son and father to the loyalty and affection of the mother continue after circumcision; both must vie for her primary loyalty. The same situation applies to sisters and wives. A man's chances of marrying a wife depend in great measure on having a younger sister or sisters, as he has a priority claim on their bridewealth. Without such sisters his chances of an early marriage, essential to the establishment of a full adult identity, are prejudiced. Without a wife he cannot maintain an independent household successfully or have children to establish his status and his line of descent.

Yet, to a large extent, the Gisu give women the same freedoms they accord to men and this results in a fairly high divorce rate, especially in the early years. Successful marriages thus depend on negotiation, especially in the most problematic areas which relate to the disposal of the products of their joint labour. Where marriage breaks down it is invariably held to be the husband's fault and here it is significant that, unlike the surrounding peoples, the Gisu do not consider that men have an automatic or 'natural' right to beat their wives. Indeed, wife-beating is subject to general condemnation and provides grounds for a wife to sue her husband in court or to divorce him.

Men's relationships with women are thus coloured by insecurity. Women are the essential help-mates but a man must vie with his father over the loyalty of his mother and with other men to retain the loyalty of his wife. We may here see the source of the repression of maternal hostility at *imbalu*. Put in a psychodynamic context, we could say (though as an anthropologist, no more than tentatively) that the idealisation of the mother is a defensive projection, consequent on the first insoluble dilemma posed to the infant who, despite his mother's inexplicable (and to the child, capricious) rejection, must continue to rely and depend upon her. Circumcision, as the final act of individuation, changes some of the terms present during weaning but not all. The boy is now presented as choosing emancipation and is 'freed', yet, in actuality, his dependence on his parents continues after circumcision. Can we see this ambiguity as being resolved, at least in part, by canalising hostile feelings towards the father? This might be one of the paradoxical implications of the rite: the boy 'saves' the mother at least partially for himself but the consequences are that he projects all his aggression onto his father and the male world which now includes himself. Autonomous manhood can be won only by means of a sacrifice but it is a sacrifice in which a man takes on responsibility for the hostility in the world.

Gender relations

Given the hostility which is seen to dominate the world of men in contrast to the world of women, this section looks further at the way in which gender relationships are depicted at *imbalu*. One of the more unusual features of *imbalu* is the way in which it valorises male gender and masculine heroism but in such a way as to draw the sexes together rather than radically opposing them. The image of complementarity is sustained. If women are weaker than men it is because they do not face the knife but this does not detract from their identification with the ritual. For example, the main myth associated with circumcision relates how the practice originated in a marriage with a woman from a neighbouring people who also circumcise women. When this woman began circumcising her daughters, the men saw that it made them 'too strong' and so started circumcising themselves instead. But if men thus checked the physical power of women, they did not take away the power altogether for *imbalu* is still held to be transmitted through women as well as men, and the myth relates how the practice spread throughout the country as a result of intermarriage.

Nevertheless, the linking of circumcision with male violence and with sexuality through the fermentation metaphor raises the question of how far, in other respects, violence is linked to sex. This theme is undoubtedly present in Bugisu, as elsewhere, but is not greatly elaborated. The equation of circumcision with virility and warriorhood is given in a common metaphor used in Kenya, that of the penis as the 'sharpened spear', trimmed for use both against other men and, of course, women. I never heard this used in Bugisu and, indeed, it could well be that the Gisu lie at the opposite extreme to some of the cultures of Kenya with their explicit gender antagonism where all sex is seen as a form of rape (see LeVine, 1959). Rather, Gisu circumcision rituals seem to proclaim a separation here by putting the emphasis on the military rather than the sexual role of men. The complementarity of the sexes and the necessity for their co-operation remains the keynote.

Circumcision does, however, provide a symbolic resource for commenting upon the relative powers of the sexes. It creates, as any complex social practice, a number of different dimensions, whose messages can be read in contrasting directions. The rites thus provide an image not only for gender asymmetry but also for gender symmetry, pulling the sexes together in so doing. For example, if one looks at the castrating aspects in the dimension of pain endured, then the Gisu directly relate circumcision to childbirth. Boys are exhorted to 'stand like a women giving birth' and the whole process, as I have outlined, puts circumcision on a par with procreation. Both men and women have experience of pain but their emotional responses to it are different. Women retain their compassion and their ability to identify with others; men are hardened by the experience and lose their compassion. In so doing, men achieve power over women. However, if one looks at circumcision in terms of blood-letting, as Bettelheim (1954) has argued, then women come out as naturally superior for, whereas it is said that men only bleed once, women are said to bleed twice. The bleeding identified here is the blood of menstruation and the blood of parturition. With respect to fertility women thus have the edge. But, again, in terms of the blood of 'spoiling', both sexes come out as equivalent; both must be 'spoilt' so they can engage in a successful and fertile adult life.

These themes played out in the ritual context give rise to its characteristic ambiguities and paradoxes. The primary one in this context is that in making a boy a man it also makes a boy *more* like a woman; not only is he identified with women 'helpers' but in the course of the ritual, he must bleed, be passive and be spoilt. Indeed, at the time of the operation the boy is essentially androgenous, combining both male and female positions, active and passive, male and castrated male. He must prove his maturity in the same way as women by being spoilt by men; the operation condensing into one symbol all the aspects of feminine maturity: bleeding, defloration, gestation and birth. If he becomes a man and not a woman it is because of what women are deemed to lack in this process – aggression. But he does not by so doing extend male mastery into the area of reproduction. The Gisu boy is made to put himself in the position of women; he does not arrogate their powers. The 'bisexuality' of the symbolism points in a rather different direction, one which again takes us back to Freudian postulate as to the original identification of child with mother and the play of both feminine and masculine identifications in the personality structures of both men and women.

If we regard circumcision as a maturation experience, a *test* of adulthood, then can we also read its symbolism as providing the materials for individual adjustment? One possibility suggested here by the psychoanalyst, Florence Begoin-Guinard, is that it might provide the opportunity for the equivalent of a transference experience.[7] Thus, we might see its symbols as allowing for the displacement of conflicts and, as in the analytic encounter, the possibility for a reworking of them in new terms. The ritual might then truly be seen to provide the occasion for personal growth: an opportunity which individuals would respond to and use differently. The promise of such an approach comes from the fact that we could then give adequate weight to both the individual and the cultural in our analyses of the rite and its effects. The fuller elaboration of such an approach is beyond the scope of this paper, but its attraction lies in its potential to develop much further the themes which are present in the ritual and the way in which these are actually handled by Gisu individuals, for example, those of sexuality and gender identity, of pain, loss and suffering, of the fusion between aggression and sexuality, of the play between destruction and creation, of choice versus constraint, and of independence versus submission.

At this point, we may return to the Oedipal dilemma and ask whether the 'spoiling' of people could be taken in a wider metaphoric way. This is the theme of the last section.

Every man a hero

Freud's writings on culture remained important to him throughout his life and he never abandoned his account of the origins of religion that he had formulated in *Totem and Taboo* (1950). Thus, he held that religion owed its origin and obsessional character to the return or unconscious memory of an act of parricide. 'Men have always known...that once upon a time they had a primeval father and killed him' (1950: 161). To expurgate the deed, appease the dead father and to allay the sense of guilt born with it, the parricidal sons began to honour the totem as the substitute for the father and renounced the fruits of their act by resigning their claim to the women of the group. Thus the primary rules of social life – the taboos on in-group murder and incest – were born. The taboos represent both the desired and the forbidden and answer to the dilemma in all of us of instinct versus the demands of social living. According to this account, circumcision is an act of sacrifice, signifying submission to the father's will, to the incest taboo, and thus to culture.

The reading of circumcision as an act of repressive socialisation is plausible in many cultural contexts, especially in those based on patriarchal gerontocracies, but does not seem to be particularly applicable to the Gisu because of the lack of a strong system of paternal authority. In turn, this raises more general problems about the application of Freudian theory with its stress on the role of the father and the paternal imaging of cultural legitimacy. This is the case whether one takes the orthodox line or, alternatively, regards the account as 'myth', that is an allegorical statement about the existential necessities for the achievement of personal autonomy and culture. Even if, after Lacan, we take it that it is the *idea* of paternal power which is important, this problem still holds for he, no less than Freud, sees the assumption of individuality, of personhood, to lie in the oedipal dynamic. Lemaire offers the following summary of Lacan's views:

> The Oedipus is the drama of a being who must become a subject and who can only do so by internalising the social rules, by entering on an equal footing into the register of the

symbolic, of Culture and of language; it is the drama of a future subject who must resolve the problem of the difference between the sexes, of the assumption of his or her own sex and of his or her unconscious drives by means of a development which presupposes the transition from natural man to man of culture.

(Lemaire, 1977: 91–92)

Oedipal conflict must happen for the individual to realise his humanity. If this is so, then circumcision should by these accounts at least provide some representation of it. At this point, I should say that it is possible to find this theme in the ritual. We can indeed interpret the rite as initiated by a symbolic killing of the father which is followed by the identification of mother and son in a sexual union. This is finally countered by the offer of a wife and reinforced by a symbolic castration as the boy faces the knife.

The first act of the circumcision ritual is, as has been mentioned earlier, the threshing of the millet which marks the boy's intent. Immediately following this, the boy and his party go into one of the father's banana plantations where the boy knocks down a bunch of bananas by smashing the stem of the tree with his bare hands. This act requires considerable strength and is met with shouts of approval. The bananas are then roasted and eaten together with a sacrificial chicken. This act is never interpreted and banana symbolism is not otherwise important in the ritual.[8] However, the destruction of the main stem may be interpreted as symbolic marker of the end of one life and the beginning of a new, represented in the basal shoots growing to replace the old (and now destroyed) stem. As such it represents both the divide at which the boy finds himself but it may also be read for messages about the father and son relationship. Indeed, the death of the old and its replacement by the new generation could hardly be more vividly depicted and, if we follow this line of reasoning, then the smashing of the stem becomes an act of symbolic parricide.

Following this, and throughout the ritual process, the mother and son become increasingly identified through the making of the circumcision beer, an act usually performed by husband and wife. Further, the image of the boy pouring water on the prepared millet could be read as an image of intercourse. For this task he must take a traditional round clay pot and fetch water from a stream or spring, carrying it back on his head without the use of a headrest. This water he then pours onto the prepared beer millet held in a much larger clay pot, immediately changing it from inert matter to a bubbling mixture. Again it is possible to read this as a representation of the boy's sexuality, with the water providing an image of semen and masculinity, while the millet represents the receptive powers of femininity. The Gisu do link men to rain and to water and women to the earth. To continue, this is followed by the boy being smeared with yeast by a senior agnate (never by his own father) together with his sisters, while the yeast is added by his mother to the brew. As has been said, this act can be taken as signifying gestation. Lastly, there is the operation itself, a 'birth' on the part of the mother, and a simultaneous death and rebirth for the son. Not implausibly, following this line of exposition, it may also be read an act of punishment inflicted by the collectivity of Gisu men on the boy for his incestuous desires.

The crucial problem with this line of interpretation is that the Gisu do not offer any commentary along these lines. To make this interpretation then we have to accept the fact of repression. However, there are evident problems for the anthropologist here because of the difference between his or her task and material and that used by the psychoanalyst. In therapeutic work, as in ritual, the dynamic adduced is that of cathartic abreaction. In order for this to be effective psychologically, the process demands an element of at least subliminal recognition, the conflict represented, as Devereux (1961) puts it, 'in a form acceptable to the ego'. It is this thesis which has frequently aroused the most anthropological hostility because of its supposed identification of cultural rituals with neurotic individual ones. Nor do we as anthropologists have access to material as to subliminal recognition. Unlike psychoanalysts where interpretative support is given in the dynamics of the analytic encounter and particularly in the fact of transference, anthropologists are more heavily reliant on the hypothetical surmise. This, it seems to me, remains an insoluble problem for this form of interpretation.

Further, even if we accept the Oedipal reading, we have some problems of interpretation. For example, in the most usual case, the boy stands for *imbalu* facing his father. Do we read this as an act of submission or an act of insubordination; the boy standing against his father and outfacing him? Or does it partake of both attitudes? Again, the problem of interpretation here, as is the problem throughout when dealing with the Gisu data, relates to the weak imaging of paternal power. If it were strong, there would be less hesitation about giving a straightforward Oedipal reading and identifying the father with authority and with tradition. But, in the Gisu case, there is a stronger argument that it is the boy and not the father who is taken to embody tradition. It is his desire to take *imbalu* which is seen as a direct inspiration and embodiment of ancestral power. Thus, he is regarded as having been 'caught' by the ancestral power of circumcision: simultaneously making manifest and submitting to the potentialities of his birth and identity. And again, the ancestral power of circumcision, like all the ancestral powers, is not identified with patriarchal authority. These powers are not fully personified but represent the continuity of ancestry, associated in a general way with the unremembered spirits of the dead, both maternal and paternal. They are not wished down by living agency but 'catch' those within their orbit.

At this point, one may take a sideways look at the process. In *Moses and Monotheism*, Freud discusses the image of the hero and its role in the creation of the idea of a high god and the particular forms of conscience recognised in both Judaism and in Christianity. Yet, his depiction of the hero or great man is also apposite here for his characterisation is strongly reminiscent of qualities all Gisu men claim for themselves. To quote from just one passage, Freud writes of the 'decisiveness of thought, the strength of will, the forcefulness of his deeds' and of 'the self-reliance and independence of the great man: his conviction of doing the right thing, which must pass into ruthlessness' (1951: 174). For Freud these characterisations belong to the picture of the archetypal father but this is not necessary. Indeed, as he mentions in another passage, 'A hero is a man who stands up manfully against his own father and in the end victoriously overcomes him' (ibid.: 18).

Gisu circumcision is a dramatic act of individuation: a boy makes himself a man. He sets himself up against his father and is circumcised standing opposite to him. In so doing he proves identity and parity with his father but, equally, he also takes on the burden of culture and commits himself bodily to it. Thus, it also presents itself as a dramatic act of conversion, attendant on the incorporation of what Fortes (1977) called 'wild youth' into the main body of society. This theme is present in the circumcision regalia whose sole purpose is said to make the boy look wild and in other imagery, such as referring to the penis at this time as *isolo*, the wild animal. From being outside the law, the boy is being made to submit to it, albeit an act represented as being of his own volition.

May we here speculate that egalitarian cultures may have a particular need for heroes which make each individual not only the bearer of culture, but a culture that is depicted as harsh and onerous? This is reminiscent of Stanner's (1963) view that Australian Aboriginal religion expresses a deep concern with a paradox central to the meaning of life, which is that the 'good life' depends upon people being willing to suffer injury. Hiatt (1975), in commenting upon this and drawing upon the work of Roheim, goes further and argues that Australian totemism and its rituals represent 'protoanalytical insights' and display significant understanding of the problems of growing up and the conditions of the unconscious. I would not want to press this claim for the Gisu but I do think it is possible to see Gisu circumcision, as outlined in the previous section, as a test for the autonomy and self-responsibility attendant upon adulthood which rests upon the individual's ability to have overcome his infantile conflicts and achieved adequate separation from the mother; thus, to have come to terms with reality and the loss and pain this involves. Almost the worst act a boy can commit during the actual operation is to call out for his mother or father. This is regarded as equally polluting as falling to the ground and likewise seen as an act of destruction, both of himself and of his family.

The father's words in Wangusa's story, 'And now do not cry anymore. You are a man', are apposite here and, in effect, summarise the whole process. The importance of the individual nature of the test is apparent in the fear of failure which runs through it. The image and threat of failure is never allowed to go away during the long build-up to the operation. While this can be seen, on the one hand, as a fairly direct process of 'battleproofing', the other side of this is to exaggerate the element of the 'test' and to highlight failure. Other peoples in Kenya, who equally insist on circumcision as a test of fortitude, do not elaborate upon the preparatory period to the same extent. Indeed, it is common for children to leave for the ceremonial sites with little or no ritual preparation and the main celebrations then follow the operation. Yet, these children are just as stoic as the Gisu and possibly even more so. For example, among the Kuria of southwest Kenya, the shamefulness of failure is considered so great that it is thought of as almost an impossibility. By contrast, a relatively large number of Gisu boys do fail. I have estimated that two or three out of ten do not stand the ordeal with the required degree of fortitude and even more try to evade it or put it off for so long that they risk being cut by force. The test of the mettle of the individual is thus certainly a very real one.

This leads me to a more general point. In other writings, I have broached the problem of how social order is maintained in systems such as that of the Gisu where the authority principle is weak. I have argued that the onus is then put on self-control. Where there are no coercive authorities to enforce the law the individual is seen as the bearer of restriction much more strongly than in authoritarian cultures. The restrictions on individual freedom are imaged in the absoluteness of taboo and this assumes the guardianship of sexual morality in Bugisu. Nevertheless, even here, morality is governed by pragmatics rather than by precept alone. The boundaries of custom, when determined through ancestral power, are changeable and each individual must, in a sense, test them out for him or herself. This makes the regulations of kinship important not only for what they explicitly prohibit but for how they should be read as general messages about the relationship of self to others. As I have argued (Heald, 1998 and Chapter Seven, this volume), these messages relate to the importance of self-denial and the necessity to exercise restraint in both sexuality and aggression.

The messages of circumcision are more ambiguous because of the power of violence which it is seen to entail. But, in undergoing *imbalu*, the boy clearly is making an unconditional statement of his place in the line of tradition and recognising its validity. In so doing, he recognises its pain and its enduring power in the marks which will be permanently inscribed on his body and in the forceful power which is now his. The 'spoiling' image is indeed apt. Circumcision, as is repeatedly said, is a bitter thing. In becoming a man, he takes on responsibility for self and, in so doing, he also takes on responsibility for the harshness of the world, a responsibility he shares with all men. To that extent every man must be a hero.

5

WITCHES AND THIEVES
Deviant motivations in Gisu society

> If a man became a habitual thief, he was looked upon as a
> public danger and was put to death publicly, sometimes by
> being beaten to death or burnt in the same way as a witch or a
> wizard. In the Gikuyu society theft and witchcraft were
> considered as very serious criminal offences.
>
> (Kenyatta, 1938: 230)

This quotation illustrates a pattern which appears to have been
common to a number of East African societies. Theft and witchcraft
were bracketed together, in that those who gained ill-repute in either
sphere were regarded as dangerous deviants and put to death.[1] Yet this
pattern, carrying with it the implications that theft and witchcraft may
be related together in other ways, has been almost entirely ignored in
the literature. This represents a significant blind spot and raises the
possibility of a bias which has directed anthropological attention to the
mystical and/or arcane beliefs and practices of other cultures and away
from the seemingly more mundane aspects and agents of misfortune.[2]
In contrast to the extensive literature on the explanatory power of
witchcraft beliefs, on the subversive nature attributed to the witch and
on accusational patterns, there is little comparable material on thieves
and thieving. The references here are tucked away in sections on
customary law and give little information on cultural stereotypes and
accusational patterns. For, by and large, theft has been treated as a self-
evident category of offence, with a direct relationship between delict
and accusation.

This assumption has neglected the implications of calling someone
a thief, an accusation as potentially damaging to the reputation of the
individual as one of witchcraft. In many societies likewise it is the
idiom for placing the individual outside the limits of customary law
and familial obligations. Nor have we, as a result, any clues as to why

'thieves' may be regarded as more of a problem in some societies rather than in others; why one might, to coin a term, have 'thief-crazes' as well as 'witch-crazes'.

From the 1960s onwards, fear of the 'kondo', armed robber, was widespread in East Africa. The national newspapers of both Kenya and Uganda carried regular bulletins of kondo attacks and the degree of public concern was clearly articulated in 1966 when robbery was made a capital offence in Uganda. In the 1970s, Amin instituted public executions for thieves, a practice which was given some publicity in Britain and seen to emphasise the barbarity of the regime. Yet, in Uganda itself, such a practice was not unpopular but seen rather as one of the more positive aspects of Amin's programme of discipline and control. It is difficult to understand such attitudes at a national level. Harsh attitudes to theft have a historical dimension and an understanding of the local cultural traditions is essential in order to grasp their generation and power.

This chapter takes up the problem with respect to the Gisu of Eastern Uganda and their attitude towards both witches and thieves during the 1960s. I argue that the accusation 'thief' would not only benefit from the type of analysis that has been seen as appropriate for witchcraft, but that in the Gisu context both types of accusations must be treated together. In Bugisu, ideas about witchcraft cannot be analysed as a self-contained explanatory system and treated in isolation from other ideas as to the sources of trouble and misfortune in the community. The semantic anthropology advocated by Crick (1976) calls for a 'recasting' of witchcraft which is capable of setting the problem in the context of differing evaluations of human action and concepts of the person which exist in other cultural settings, a form of analysis which could evidently embrace both witchcraft and theft. On both counts we need to widen our schema of relevance.

Gisu attitudes to witches and thieves

There are a number of similarities between witchcraft (*bulosi*) and theft (*bubifi*) in Gisu society. One can start with the fact that the killing of both witches and thieves is not only regarded as justifiable (as, for example, is the case with killing an adulterer *in flagrante delicto*) but positively acclaimed as a service to the community. Nor is the threat of such killing in any way idle. In Bugisu, it is a common sight to see a party of men, armed with sticks and knobkerries, on the tracks of a thief. Once found, he can expect extremely, extremely harsh treatment, being roped and then beaten with every passer-by lending a hand, despite the prosecutions for manslaughter that the assailants then risk in the Ugandan courts. As with the Kikuyu, the method of killing witches is different, the favoured means being to fire the thatch of the suspect's house at night and then spear him as he attempts to escape. When I first arrived in Bugisu in 1965 these killings tended to be done by *ad hoc* groups, but in the late 1960s organised groups of vigilantes developed in all areas of Bugisu.[3] Their popular appeal rested firmly on the fear that witchcraft and theft generated and the promise made to usher in a new era of Gisu justice. The problem, as the Gisu saw it, is illustrated by the following quote by a vigilante leader, who had come to set up a vigilante group in a nearby area.

> We are the vigilantes and are trying to bring law and order into this area. Where we live there are no longer any thieves and people can leave their houses without worry. We leave everything around – cows, goats, clothes – and when we return they are still there. But you are still suffering. Look at that person there whom they have bewitched! He is going to die! And that one over there! Is there anyone here who is not afraid for his life? We have come because we want there to be peace everywhere. So those who say they are fearful of their own lives or those of their friends, raise your hands and tell us of the witches and thieves.

So who were the witches and thieves who were denounced at trials such as these? In one way there was no great problem for their identity was the subject of consensus. So much so that one of the first things I learnt as a novice anthropologist were the categories of dangerous person, whom if I were wise I would treat with scrupulous civility and avoid as far as possible.

Yet this apparent visibility of offenders raises its own problems. Why were they so easily recognised? What characteristics marked them out? The point to be made here is that there is frequently little objective evidence to link a particular person with a theft in Bugisu as is generally assumed by anthropologists in dealing with witchcraft. I do not mean to imply by this that no-one steals – indeed petty-pilfering is rife – but that the culpability of a particular individual is by no means always obvious. The density of settlement together with the rather amorphous nature of social life ensures that whenever something goes missing a great number of people could be the potential culprits. The same, of course, is true of witchcraft; there is rarely any lack of possible suspects. But situational allegation is not really the point at issue.

Indeed, everyone has their own, essentially private, circle of enemies and practically everyone comes under some suspicion of resorting to witchcraft or theft as a way of avenging themselves on those enemies at some point in their lives. But relatively few people have their names promulgated as 'thieves' or 'witches'. For such an appellation implies rather more than that the individual concerned has stolen or bewitched: it is a fuller assessment of character. In the case of thieves, the appellation 'thief' is synonymous with 'bad lot', a wastrel, or a troublemaker. Thus a 'thief' is as much a person thought likely to take to stealing as one who has actually been caught doing so. When the Gisu then talk of thieves or witches they imply an ultimate dispositional base from which such behaviour can be seen to spring.

One important concept here is that of *lirima*. Those who gain reputations as thieves or witches are thought of as in the grip of excessive *lirima*. *Lirima* is not in itself an anti-social quality. On the contrary, it is regarded as an essential quality in a man. All men must have the force of character it implies to go through the rites of circumcision and to stand up for their rights in everyday life thereafter. Yet *lirima* is not seen as a constant facet of the personality, rather it is an effervescent quality which 'bubbles up' in a man, and can then dictate his thoughts and actions. *Lirima* in this context is identified as an actual physical symptom, the lump in the throat which develops when a man is intensely angry. In this form, then, *lirima* implies uncontrollable anger or resentment, awakened in the normal man in limited and specific circumstances. In thieves and confirmed witches it is, however, believed to be a more consistent feature and, since their spleen is uncontrollable, it is seen to be indiscriminate as well. Such men are deemed dangerous to the community at large, however trivial the actual offences with which they are charged.

This vernacular psychology directs attention to some accusational limitations. The most important is that thieves (*babifi*) are always men. Women are never considered thieves. That is, although I came across cases where women stole, usually from a husband, a brother or a lover, they were never regarded as incorrigible thieves and were certainly never killed on such a pretext.[4] This is consistent with the Gisu belief that women cannot feel *lirima* but only the weaker emotion *libuba*. Likewise in children the capacity is believed to be undeveloped. The situation is slightly different with witchcraft for women are believed to have access to certain forms, though generally only the weaker types consistent with their weaker powers, though this does not imply that it is any the less feared.

Nevertheless, theft and witchcraft are *not* synonymous as accusations. While they are alike in that they can be seen as related to a similar dispositional base, they are in fact aimed at different sections of the population. Theft is an accusation which is aimed predominantly at young men. This is amply illustrated by the court records for the period between 1960 and 1966. Of the 375 homicide cases indicted before the District Court during that time 97 (26 per cent) of these were thief-killings and the overwhelming majority (86 per cent) of these thieves were aged between twenty and thirty-nine. In contrast, witchcraft accusations are aimed at the old. In the court sample, witch-killings are under-represented and form a numerically less significant total, some thirteen cases, but in all these the suspected witch was over forty-five years old.[5] This pattern is consistent with Gisu beliefs in that the power or capacity (*bunyali*) to indulge in witchcraft is an attribute of age. A person's *bunyali* (related to the verb, *xunyala*, to be able) is believed to grow with age, not only increasing their wisdom, but also any capacity to feel anger and any bent towards witchcraft. Again, *bunyali* operates as a dispositional or inherent attribute and discriminates between men and women, for women's power, their *bunyali*, is held to be always inferior to men's.

The homicide statistics given above point to a strong pattern of intergenerational conflict and one which has been emphasised by Jean la Fontaine (1960; 1967). In her writings on parricide, La Fontaine relates it to the 'competition between the generations for the control of the means of acquiring prestige' (1960: 109). It is worth noting that in the 1960s with a far greater overall rate of homicide (thirty-two per 100,000 as compared with seven per 100,000 at the time of La Fontaine's study) parricide as such formed a less significant aspect of the total homicide statistics. La Fontaine's data for the years between 1948–54 revealed seven cases of parricide out of a total of sixty-seven (10 per cent) while mine give eight out of 375 (2 per cent). Nevertheless, I also see the system of property transmission as crucial in this case to an understanding of accusations of witchcraft and theft. Not only because accusational processes can be seen as generated, in part, by intergenerational conflict, but also because of the effect the inheritance system has, in the present economic situation in Bugisu, of creating categories of impoverished adult men.

There is a large body of literature on accusational patterns involving witchcraft with the witch located in marginal or structurally ambiguous positions. In East and Central Africa, the focus has been on accusational processes in the context of competition for village headships, related to the developmental cycle of these residential groups (Mitchell 1956; Turner 1957; Middleton 1960; Marwick 1965). The 'witches' have been seen as caught in an inevitable political process unable to achieve power or unable to maintain it. Similarly, in Bugisu, I see both witches and thieves as casualties or failures in the system. However, I argue that these accusations are not associated with the development cycle of groups but rather related to the life cycle of individuals and with competition for basic economic resources. At certain points in their lives Gisu men become vulnerable to accusation if they fail to gain or maintain control over sufficient resources to establish their position as adult men.

La Fontaine has written that in Bugisu, 'inegalities are the more glaring for the ideal of equality' (1963: 216). It is not inequality itself which I see as at issue but the insistence on a specific model of manhood, an irreducible basis, which requires material independence. A man, by definition, possesses the capability for *lirima* which, as a legitimate mode of self-assertion, can only be exercised by an autonomous man who, in defending his rights, has no reason to envy others. Where this ceases to be the case the individual may sharply lose social credibility, his motivations suspect, his powers feared. This places peculiar stress on the young and the old, just as in modern condition, anyone who meets in the course of life with ill luck or disease is placed in a situation where all is risked.

The accusational setting

Gisu settlement is continuous: there are no discrete bounded communities at any territorial level. While the Gisu have a fairly elaborate patrilineal lineage and clan organisation, lineage identity is a weak principle at the neighbourhood level with little factionalism along the lines of lineage cleavage. Rather Gisu social organisation is characterised by a division and spread of loyalties with each individual being the pivot of his or her own network of social relations. Outside the narrow span of the agnatic lineage (2–3 generations in depth), with a dispersed membership a man's strongest loyalties are to his brothers-in-law, maternal kin and age mates. One corollary of this is that there is no feuding pattern and, indeed, with such a lack of corporate commitment, no marked vengeance-killing pattern either. That is, kinsmen do not avenge each other's deaths nor do they recognise an unequivocal responsibility to protect each other during life.

A dominant theme in Gisu life is the stress on the autonomy of the individual and the right of a man to control his own affairs without interference from others. This individualistic emphasis is important in understanding the standards Gisu demand of their menfolk and the intricate connection which exists between the evaluation of character and individual achievement. Throughout, the stress is upon the personal qualities which allow some men to succeed in life where others fail. This is brought out forcibly in the circumcision rites which bridge the gulf between boyhood (*businde*) and manhood (*busetsa*). Most boys are circumcised when they are between sixteen and twenty-four years old, though the range is somewhat greater than this. The boy himself chooses the exact year and, in theory, no-one can force a boy to be circumcised, a point reiterated as a boy's senior kinsmen prepare him for the operation. The strength to endure the ordeal with courage must come from himself; if his heart is not in it then no one can help him. The boys' songs as they dance in the months before the rituals glory in the independence of their choice and their own determination to 'face death'.

The rites of circumcision symbolise the removal of the boy from jural identification with his father to a position of his own in the community. After circumcision he takes his place as an equal among men, eligible for all the privileges associated with adulthood. He may now drink beer with other men but, more importantly, he must now set up his own household. After circumcision his father should provide him with the resources necessary to make him economically independent: land and the cattle necessary for bridewealth. The allocation of these resources forms the basis of the young man's wealth and he must thereafter expand such resources largely through his own efforts and those of his wife. Indeed, the evaluation accorded individuals is largely indistinguishable from their wealth and manifest success. Poverty, like wealth, is seen to be the result of individual qualities and indigence is judged harshly. The feckless wander around instead of cultivating, spend their money on beer instead of caring for their family. For such men there is only contempt.

But individual enterprise is not the only factor which determines wealth. For the initial allocation of resources a man is totally dependent upon his father and, in turn, upon his father's relative wealth, the number of other sons he must provide for, the number of cattle received in bridewealth from his daughters and last, but by no means least, upon his father's generosity. It is on this issue of the allocation of basic items of wealth that the values placed on autonomy and self-reliance run directly counter to the actual fact of a man's dependence upon his father and more generally upon his senior kinsmen.

La Fontaine is undoubtedly correct in seeing the father-and-son relationship at the crucial intersection of, on the one hand, ideals of competitive equality among adults and, on the other, genealogically ascribed authority and patrilineal transmission of property (La Fontaine, 1967). The inherent conflict of interests in the relationship and the ambivalence of sentiment this generates is not bounded by an absolute stress on filial piety, supported by symbols of the father's ritual authority. Nor are the roles of father and son separated by ritual avoidance as is found in some societies where, as in Bugisu, the son may be seen to abrogate his father's wealth and position. Rather, the ideal is one of mutuality; the father nurturing his son, preparing the way for his safe and successful circumcision and providing him with property thereafter. In return, the son should be respectful and obedient, honouring his father. Nevertheless, it is recognised that the relationship frequently falls short of the ideal, developing into a polarisation of mutually hostile interests. The dangers resulting from such alienation are readily drawn as the following statement by an elder in Central Bugisu shows:

> If the child is troublesome and disregards his father's words then he belittles any gift his father makes, saying it is not enough. He wants to get everything from his father and cares nothing for him. His father may say 'Why do you quarrel like this with me all the time when I have given you land and cattle to marry a wife?' Such fathers and sons keep on fighting for the son is after his father's last cow – and for that they kill. Or the son wants the land which the father's old wife is still cultivating – and for that they kill.

Goodwill is recognisably hard to maintain as fathers procrastinate in order to preserve for a few more years their wealth and position in the community, and sons press their claims with growing impatience. For while common sense and the weight of approved customary behaviour require that a son should bide his time and be a dutiful son, many pressures militate against such a subservient position. The tangible aspect of full adult status is to be economically self-sufficient and this is the crux. A man without bridewealth cannot marry and without a wife he cannot maintain a household successfully. He is forced either to demean himself with 'women's work' or to rely on another household for food, a cause of considerable resentment on both sides. It is bachelors who tend to attract accusations; of violence (*butemu*), brawling (*bulomani*), inciting other people to anger (*uwe kamaya*), adultery (*buweyani*) and, above all, of theft (*bubifi*). They are regarded as general nuisances, *batambisi*, this noun deriving from the verb *xatamba* 'to be without'.

This is not to say that only bachelors get accused of serious offences but that the system of evaluation encourages this. This relates, in part, simply to plausibility, so that any sign of *lirima* draws unfavourable attention. Their thieving relates to the fact that they have no visible means of subsistence; their adulteries to the lack of a wife. Failure to gain or keep a wife in particular (and marriage in the early years tends to be unstable) is often taken as symptomatic of the individual being 'spoilt', and thus unable to persevere in the normal pursuits of adulthood. Indeed, bachelors are unable to fully participate in adult occupations and for reasons which can only be indicated here, the longer a man remains a bachelor, the more likely he is effectively to lose his inheritance rights. The Gisu proverb, 'something which is spoilt goes on spoiling itself' is indeed prophetic and underlines the fate of many bachelors and the attitudes adopted towards them.

This can be briefly illustrated with the case of Mwayafu who was beaten to death as a thief at the age of twenty. The following account was given by his father's brother who had reared Mwayafu since his real father died fifteen years before:

> Mwayafu was a troublesome youth and never wanted to settle down to anything or to cultivate. I gave him land but he just sold it and then I refused him saying how could I give him more land just to sell? He only wanted to drink beer with his friends and everyone complained of little things missing from their compounds. He took everything, chickens, clothes, money and blankets. I said 'Papa, why do you do these things and make your kin angry?' but he disregarded me and began to abuse me until we quarrelled and he cut me with his knife.
>
> Soon afterwards we were all mourning at a funeral when a man came from another area saying that he had traced the footsteps of the thief who had stolen all his clothes to our place. We were very angry and went to Mwayafu's house and tied him up and began to beat him.

The portrayal of Mwayafu's character falls into a conventional pattern. The Gisu see the position of such men as largely self-induced; it is a man's own actions which precipitate the harsh action later meted out to him. Such men are deemed oblivious to the reasonable arguments of their kin and may turn even on those who have cared for them. Moreover, the fault is firmly located in the psychological make-up of the individuals. Their actions are made explicable only by evoking the concept of *tsinje*, an inherent quality which manifests itself in acts which are not only self-defeating but make them a danger to those around them. Their *lirima* is not directed towards the normal activities of manhood but against themselves and, ultimately, against the community at large. This attitude in turn justifies repudiation by their close kin, whom it also absolves from any moral responsibility for their predicament. No man is held at fault for denying resources to a wastrel son. In such instances the accusation of theft can be seen to be the cultural idiom for the repudiation of responsibility for the individual.

It is important to stress, however, that there are *no* acceptable roles for wifeless men in Gisu society. Those that are tolerated in the community achieve adaptations to their position, which although deviant, define them as more or less harmless. One such man was Maboni:

> In 1969, Maboni was thirty-six and lived in a make-shift shelter of plantain leaves, going out each day to cut down firewood which he sold to buy the maize meal on which he lived. He had constructed a somewhat rickety ladder to enable him to climb into the taller trees and lop off those branches out of reach of the women who are forbidden to climb trees. Apart from that, he was rarely seen around the neighbourhood for he lived as a recluse, neither visiting nor visited by the fifteen members of his lineage segment who lived nearby. For the most part he stayed around his shelter or wandered off into another neighbourhood when he had enough money to buy beer. His kinsmen called him by the nickname, Walele, which means literally one who is silent or who talks nonsense. This name in part related to Maboni's speech which was thick and slurred and hardly intelligible. Yet his kin also thought the name apt for other reasons: his wild and rugged appearance, dressed in rags with uncombed hair and his neglect of all personal cleanliness, for he was reputed never to wash or to clean his shelter. Nor did he care to do any of the normal work of a man for he made no attempt to cultivate his small plot of land. Nor did he chase women. People said that he had never shown any interest in women and was probably impotent.

There were other men of this kind whose lifestyles, as Maboni's, seemed to revolve around the avoidance of all situations where they might be regarded as competitors for basic resources or where they might run the risk of acrimony from their kin and neighbours. Such lifestyles have fundamental consequences for those concerned, for to be convincing they must be absolute, absolute in their rejection of the basic values associated with manhood and any chance of achieving the resources which could improve their status in the area. Nevertheless, they still run the risk of being convenient scapegoats for minor misfortunes and when bunches of plantain went missing it was often Maboni who was suspected. However, his life was in much less danger than those whose frustrations with their position led them to open violence against those they blamed for their misfortunes.

It is this question of blame that relates directly to certain witchcraft beliefs. Witchcraft, especially cursing, holds the key to a wide variety of personal failings which are for the Gisu so intimately linked – infertility, failure to get or to keep a wife, lingering illness, indolence, theft and violent behaviour. For cursing is believed to change a man's heart and thus his attitude to the world, turning an industrious youth into a wastrel, doomed to failure in all aspects of adult life. In contrast to some African societies where cursing or invoking the ancestors is seen, at least in certain circumstances, as the legitimate prerogative of the old, in Bugisu it is regarded as the most heinous use of supernatural power (*bulosi*). Far from supporting the authority of the old, inducing obedience and respect, it tends to underline the structural hostility between the generations, with the old seen as ever tempted to abuse their ritual powers and bring destruction to their line. Only the senior generation have the power to curse (*citsubo*), and in so doing are believed to put themselves in league with the dead against the living. They invoke the ghosts of the recently dead, the *bamakombe*, who are seen not only as resentful of the fact of death but still prey to the malice and ill-will which followed them in life. They attack because they 'want to eat', appearing in dreams to state their demands. On one level then, their motive is always 'greed', as indeed is that of the cursers who, like the ghosts, put their own selfish interest over and above the wellbeing of their descendants. If the ghosts want sacrifices or new tombstones, the cursers likewise want feasts and gifts. Since fear of cursing permeates all senior–junior relationships children are persistently warned to give their last cent to a senior person who asks for it.

Significantly, it is the time when a boy stands on the threshold of adult life that such dangers are believed to be most acute. Circumcision is a focus of danger for the initiate for while his success is linked to his personal courage, he is also susceptible to dangers beyond his control. The beliefs emphasise the boy's dependence on the senior generation on whom he must rely for protection just as they reiterate their potential malevolence. Before circumcision the good and bad luck the boy has experienced are a product of the forces aimed at his parents and their ability to protect him. Thereafter, he will be a target for such forces in his own right and responsible for defending his own family. What befalls him at the time of his circumcision, however, depends both upon his own qualities and upon the goodwill of the senior generation who must undertake his ritual protection.

Failure in any number of areas here can bring harm to the initiate at the time of the operation and, more importantly, can affect his chances of a successful life as an adult. When a man finds it difficult to marry, his children die, or he himself becomes weak and ill or he takes to wandering and theft, then it is frequently in the maleficent powers of those who claimed to be protecting him at the time of his circumcision that both he and others will seek the cause of his misfortune. Serious accusations of cursing thus cling to those intangible situations where a man feels that his chances in life are not only being hindered by the overt selfishness of the senior generation, but that they are attempting to subvert the course of his life through supernatural means as well. Killing in such circumstances is considered legitimate.

To summarise, two prominent accusational patterns have been outlined: those of theft aimed at indigent young men, and those of cursing which are generated by their dissatisfaction with their position and aimed at those they hold responsible. One other form of accusation relates similarly to the individual life cycle, to the problems faced by older men who become impoverished as a result of the inheritance system which obliges them to distribute the greater part of their resources among their adult sons.

Apart from cursing (*citsubo*), the evil eye (*ifumu*) (winking) and night dancing (*bubini*), there are about fifteen major different categories of 'medicine' which 'catch' their victims in a variety of ways. These beliefs, in turn, are tied to an elaborate aetiology of disease with each variety of witchcraft (*bulosi*) related to specific symptoms. It is further believed that a witch may have access to any number of these according to his or her powers which depend in part on age and sex. The most powerful forms of *bulosi* are the prerogative of old men since women are believed to have neither the power (*bunyali*) nor the motivation as implied by *lirima* to utilise the more lethal forms of witchcraft.

The motive behind the use of witchcraft is usually detailed as anger, greed, envy or revenge. In this respect witchcraft is looked upon as a fairly straightforward means of aggression which, depending on the circumstances, can be legitimate. Indeed, by extension, *bulosi* may be used in speech to refer to any act of violent aggression. However, some witches are regarded not only as *balosi* but attributed with a power called *liroko* which sets them in a different motivational category. In part, such an appellation is a matter of degree, for some people take umbrage more easily than others. In its ultimate form, however, it implies that their actions are not susceptible to rational interpretation. In terms of the normal range of emotions that people feel they are 'motiveless'. Such people are believed to put themselves in league not with the ghosts as do the cursers but with the spirits of the unincorporated dead, the *were*, those of the childless, the hunchbacked and the crippled whose life forces are not inherited but doomed to forever haunt the bush. While *liroko* is not in itself tied to the use of any specific witchcraft technique (all may be called *buroki*), it does have its typical manifestations and, in old men, it is evident particularly in *bubini* or night-dancing.

This is a unique category of male witchcraft in several ways. The night-dancer is not believed to deal in medicines but harms simply by the act of dancing. He goes out naked at night and, accompanied by his familiars, owls and wild cats, dances around his neighbours' houses. He also has his own song – a song which any child can repeat, giggling as he does so:

> Am I a night dancer, a night dancer?
> Do I mend it! Do I ruin it?
> aa aa aa

The very words of this song suggest the ambivalent attitude Gisu have to this form of witchcraft. On the one hand, it is thought that night-dancers only want to frighten others and the harm they do is never of a very serious nature. Indeed, during the daylight hours the idea of such witches holds little terror. An adult man will scoff at them, inviting the night-dancers to come and dance outside his house for at least they will frighten away the thieves and all he will have in the morning are aching joints or perhaps a slight fever. Moreover, they can easily be dealt with. In order to prevent the actions of other witches proving fatal ritual specialists must be consulted, but night-dancers can be tackled by the individual. A good beating is considered sufficient to deter them. Yet, just as the night-dancers are the only really fantastic figures in Gisu witchcraft mythology, so too are their punishments. First one must catch one's night-dancer. This is fairly easy as they dance with their buttocks bumping against the door. So one quietly undoes the hinges from the inside and, hey presto, in he falls. Then, there is a choice of punishments. He might be speared up the anus or under the tongue with the shoot of a banana leaf, after which he will go away and silently die. When old men die it is frequently rumoured that they have been killed by such means.

Indeed, there is a sense in which all old men carry the presumption of *bubini* in much the same way as bachelors do of theft. The old are definitionally powerful, but this power is not that of active manhood, which slips away through their disposal of their resources as well as by infirmity or illness, reducing them again to a state of dependence. The old gain little respect as elders; their power, their *bunyali*, lies in their control of knowledge (*kamaxura*), a knowledge which implies witchcraft. Housed and fed on sufferance, their every complaint is seen to carry the threat of it. It is in terms of this pervasive fear that the attitudes to night-dancers have their place. Despite the apparent ease of ritual murder, the sentiment that night-dancers deserve outright death is uppermost.

That the old are indeed frequently killed can again be referred to the homicide statistics for the District. In terms of absolute numbers more young men are killed. This is, however, a function of the age structure of the population and, if the figures are converted into rates for each age group, then it is apparent that the chance of being a victim of homicide in fact increases dramatically with age, viz. 46.7 per 100,000 for men between fifteen and twenty-nine, 80.5 for men between thirty and forty-four but 132.8 for men older than this.[6] A contrast can be drawn with those accused of homicide. The proportion of accused rises abruptly after the age of fifteen and reaches a peak in the age group twenty-five to twenty-nine, one quarter of all accused being of this age. Thereafter, the percentages decrease with equal abruptness. Thus, whereas the chance of being killed in Bugisu increases with age, that of being an offender decreases after the age of thirty, giving strong support to the accusational dynamic outlined in this chapter.

Conclusion

I have concentrated on cultural values and the presentation of 'deviant' types, very much as the Gisu see them. I have also indicated the major structural and economic factors which underline the dominant accusational patterns. To summarise, economic wealth and control is in the hands of mature men between the ages of thirty and fifty; that is, those who have achieved their inheritance and not yet been obliged to reallocate their wealth to their descendants. Allegations of witchcraft and theft are aimed not at such people but at the unfortunate or impoverished who lack sufficient resources to maintain themselves independently. This, as has been indicated, is most likely to occur at the two extreme ends of the adult life-cycle. In turn, such accusations can be used to assert claims and restrict access to scarce resources.

One further query can be dealt with. The Gisu saw their society as increasingly harassed by thieves and witches. What credence can one give this perception? In terms of the accusational process outlined, it would in fact seem a realistic assessment of the situation for there was increasing pressure on the basic resource, land. Land pressure is a notoriously difficult thing to measure. Nevertheless, the overall density in Bugisu, together with a 30 per cent increase in the population between the censuses of 1959 and 1969, attest to its possible severity. Certainly land-holdings are becoming increasingly fragmented and many men, to my knowledge, owned less land than met their subsistence needs. Added to this, the thorough-going commercialisation of the economy, stemming from the success of cash cropping and the differential rewards from wage labour, is tending towards the creation of classes of rich and poor. Land and labour are both marketable commodities. On a day-to-day basis all services between men are on a strictly cash basis and as much land is transferred by sale as it is by inheritance. There are, as a result of this, few checks today to prevent a poor man losing all the land he relies on for livelihood. In times of misfortune, such as death or illness in the family, famine or simply to raise tax money, a poor man might have to realise his only capital asset, his land. Growing land shortage in the District is thus associated with insecurity of tenure for the poorer sections of the community.

In exploring a similar problem involving acute land shortage among the Chagga of Tanzania, Sally Moore interprets disputes and the ranking processes contained within them as 'part of a desperate elimination context in which the community must slough off members to survive (1975: 113). Again, certain structurally-placed individuals are most vulnerable, in this case the 'middle-sons' who are least favoured by the inheritance system. In commenting on the moral conflicts raised by this process she writes that some of the pain 'of rejecting a brother is ameliorated if he can be identified as a bad character who is at least partially to blame for his own plight, as a person who is morally inadequate' (ibid.: 136). The fate of such men varies. Among the Chagga, they are forced off the land to become the unskilled, and often unemployed, of the towns. Among the Gisu a similar process is observable though, as is evident, a considerable proportion meet a violent end, becoming part of the rising crime statistics of East Africa.

As Radcliffe-Brown (1940) pointed out long ago, the crime at issue is not the commission of any single offence but that of being a 'bad lot', as he termed it. In this chapter, I have been concerned to indicate the more important concepts – *lirima, tsinje, liroko* – which inform and comprise such evaluations of character among the Gisu. What is significant is that they are seen as dispositional attributes which, as such, are inherent, unalterable and irremediable. Reform in such cases ceases to be a possibility. It is not that killing is justified because the offence in itself is great, but it is justified because the individual is regarded as a degenerate who has turned his back on normality and for whom there is no other remedy. It is only in such terms that killing over the theft of a bunch of bananas or a single root of cassava becomes as likely as killing over the theft of cattle. *Tsinje* is a critical idea here and it is used in contexts that oppose it to respect and order, *lukoosi*, the mode of harmonious and proper living as a member of the community. When faced with a breakdown in the community it was *lukoosi* that the vigilantes sought to impose not only by the direct expedient of killing witches and thieves but by imposing often elaborate rules of discipline upon the Gisu neighbourhoods. The vigilantes were generally known as *banalukoosi* (men of order), their targets and victims were identified with *tsinje* (disorder).

In that branch of psychology known as attribution theory there is a considerable body of literature on the assessment of motive. Attribution theorists (such as Heider 1958; Jones and Nisbet 1971; Kelley 1971; and Shaver 1975) suggest that one of the most powerful tools used in the explanation of behaviour is to see it as a product of personal dispositions or traits. *Dispositional* attributions coexist with *environmental* attributions where behaviour is seen to result from situational constraints. However, on the basis of experimental work, it has been suggested that concentration on another's disposition provides a more compelling evaluative mode since dispositional attribution not only provides a rationale for the behaviour under review but also provides a basis for predicting future behaviour. In other words it integrates past and present information about the person with a coherent scheme of 'personality'. As Shaver writes: 'the perceiver's motivation to engage in an attribution is a need to simplify his perceptual world by *explaining* the present and past behaviour of others and by *predicting* with some degree of accuracy what those people are likely to do in the future' (1975: 29–30). Such attributions then have important cognitive functions, an aspect of the attempt to control the human world and render it predictable. Their moral implications in the form of labelling and stereotyping have been more fully explored in the sociology of deviance by the symbolic interactionist or labelling theorists.[7]

Garfinkel (1956), for example, talks of the deviant as a 'motivational type' as opposed to a 'behavioural type', when the former is judged in terms of what the group holds to be the ultimate grounds or reasons for his performance.

The switch from one evaluative mode to another is evidently crucial to understanding processes of accusation and their effects at the interpersonal level. In Bugisu, one can recognise both types of attribution and their differential applications in day-to-day life. Whereas the aggressive acts of most men are seen as isolated instances, relative to the situation in which they occurred, the behaviour of others is judged according to their disposition which makes any situational attribution with its possibility of extenuating circumstances (understandable if not appropriate behaviour) largely irrelevant. In such a way an impressive dossier of the misdeeds of certain members of the community can be presented and further publicised in a way inconceivable for others. The deviance of such men is total. Such attribution relates to economic status. In turn, this depends on more general normative ideas. At one level, what is at issue is the state of manhood itself. In Goffman's (1968) usage, the Gisu have strong identity norms, holding out uncompromising standards for their menfolk. The stereotype of what is normal in a man is highly valued culturally and given added impact in the circumcision ceremonials which give formal admittance to adult status. By casting those who fail to live up to such a standard in a distinctly inimical mould, the Gisu have been able to preserve an image of Gisu manhood and all the connotations this has for Gisu culture at a time when it is under threat. The price paid for such a strategy is perhaps self-evident.

6

DIVINATORY FAILURE
Gisu diviners and the problem of doubt

'When it kills you, then you will know it,' runs a Gisu proverb, and it may be used to point to three themes present in Gisu divination. First, that it is retrospective: it seeks to uncover or reveal the causes of misfortune in the present history of the person. As a tradition it is thus backward- and not forward-looking; it is one that makes little use of prophecy or prediction. Second, Gisu divination operates exclusively in situations of personal danger and uncertainty and, in my experience, it reproduces and confirms this view. 'When it kills you, then you will know it' implies rather more than that death is the only certainty, for it involves the idea that the person cannot fully know what he or she is up against until finally beaten. Divination, it is true, aims to reveal this – to depict the range, strength and malignancy of the influences at work upon the individual – but, as will be outlined, authoritative pronouncements are rare. This connects with the last point, which is that divination operates essentially in the private sphere and, at the time I was in Bugisu in the late 1960s, had no public role. Diviners were not priests; they were not called in to officiate at family rituals, at the *rites de passage* of birth, circumcision and death. Nor did they gain a following as renowned healers or play any role in wider community affairs.

Indeed, it is this very insignificance that I want to concentrate on. The anthropological literature has tended to discuss divination and divinership only when it has been seen to play a notable (and positive) role in the transformation of social relationships, whether these have been seen in repetitive cyclic terms as, for example, in the work of Turner (1957; 1967; 1975) or in the transformation of society (for example, Parkin, 1968; Lan, 1985). This concentration on the prominence of diviners leads us to overlook their relative social invisibility elsewhere. Yet perhaps we may gain some insight into the rise of prophets and charismatic healers by considering the other side of this story and looking at the multitude of very humble practitioners plying their trade. What is the social role of divination here? What areas of experience does divination serve to express and articulate? How does their social insignificance relate to the nature of their apparent 'power'? These are the questions I want to explore.

They link with one further theme, which is the degree of credibility that divination commands. Since Evans-Pritchard's (1937) account of Azande witchcraft a degree of scepticism in African attitudes to divination has formed part of our standard set of expectations. Evans-Pritchard was clearly surprised to find a considerable body of quizzical opinion among the Azande, and reports that most of his acquaintances 'believed that there are a few reliable practitioners, but that the majority are quacks' (1937: 185). Further, the Azande were often cynical about the tricks performed by witch-doctors during their dramatic and theatrical seances and clearly understood the possibility – and even likelihood – of fraud. So why, he asks, 'does not common sense triumph over superstition' (ibid.: 193)? The elegance of his answer has become basic to understanding the problem ever since. Scepticism, he showed, was part of the pattern of belief: directed at the particular practitioner, it in no way challenges the premises of the belief system itself, which emerge not only unscathed but reinforced, as the possibilities of such fraudulence serve to explain away its failures.

While I do not wish to challenge the argument in itself, one consequence has been to make this area essentially unproblematic, with attention deflected away. African scepticism is seen as part of a more generally conservative bias: its function is to support the status quo of belief. Thus it has not been examined as a variable, more typical of some social situations than of others. If we are to explore the character of African scepticism more fully, I would argue that we should not see it as an aspect of some supposed universal faculty but enquire into the social bases of knowledge. We should not ask, as Evans-Pritchard did, about how belief is sustained despite the presence of scepticism – why it is that common sense does not win out against mystical thinking – but more generally what it is about the nature of these beliefs and their situational context which *encourages* scepticism. I suspect that it is not useful to explore this issue in terms of the rationality question or the 'truth' of belief systems. If we are to draw a comparison with modern attitudes, of greater significance might be the organisation and differentiation of knowledge and its relationship to power. In this context I propose to look at Gisu practices to see how scepticism can be related to the relative power of diviner and client and to the nature of the knowledge involved. I will suggest that diagnostic systems used by societies such as the Gisu encourage an agnostic attitude in a way in which those of the modern West do not.

Gisu diviners

In Gisu society, diviners are individuals who have been 'caught' by the ancestral power of divination (*bufumu*) and set up in practice as a consequence. In any area there are very many of them and they form part of an intricate system of part-time specialists dealing with sickness and misfortune. The Gisu have a fairly elaborate aetiology of disease, so that symptoms suggest the appropriate causal agency and thus the means of cure and counteraction. Yet, while all illness and misfortune suggests an 'outside' agency – in various forms of witchcraft and cursing, in the intervention of ancestral ghosts or possession by ancestral powers – it is not necessarily important to identify the source of the trouble positively. Minor illnesses – colds, fevers, cuts, sores, aches and diarrhoea – may be directly treated by simplistic and other remedies, acting either to alleviate the symptoms directly (as with Western medicines and herbal potions) or to neutralise lesser forms of sorcery. Some medicines – for colds and fever, for example – are widely known, while others are known by individuals who offer treatment in return for payment. Some of these set themselves up as regular 'doctors', *bakanga*, offering a range of cures and protective devices. Of these some are *bamomoli*, who claim the ability to 'draw out' sorcery substance from the stomach of the afflicted. These specialists are the first line of defence in terms of illness, and it is only when such means fail that people will usually consider resorting to diviners (*bafumu*). Expense, in itself, cannot be seen as the critical deterrent here, as the cost of an initial consultation was usually 3s., comparable if not cheaper than seeking alternative remedies. Rather, it is severity which prompts people to seek out diviners in the hope of both establishing a diagnosis – that is, the causal agency involved – and invoking more powerful forms of counteraction.

Diviners claim special powers by virtue of having been caught by the ancestral power of divination (*bufumu*), which gives them direct communication with the ancestral world and access also to distinctive forms of counteraction. All may attempt to interpret the wishes of the ancestral ghosts (*bamakombe*) or the ancestral spirits (*basambwa*) and their associated powers (*kimisambwa*), while some also claim powers to counteract sorcery. Of these latter, some are recognised sorcery seekers, known as *balyuli*, who 'smell out' sorcery substances buried along the paths or in the compound or hidden in the thatch of houses. Others are known to practise more direct forms of vengeance sorcery. And, while there is no clear line of division between the people who know one or two medicines, simples for particular illnesses, and more widely reputed healers, the same may be said of the diviners. The power of divination (together with the power of circumcising) is probably the most widely distributed of Gisu ancestral powers. Thus in any area many people are known to have been caught by it. Rather fewer tend actually to practise as diviners.

Nevertheless, there are very many of them, with probably equal numbers of men and women.[1] The sexual division is marked generally by the forms of counteraction they practise. Women, whose powers in respect of witchcraft are deemed less than men's, rarely undertake sorcery eradication, counteraction or vengeance sorcery. However, they may become reputed for their divining skills and officiate at rituals to accommodate or naturalise a person with the ancestral powers which are troubling him or her. Male diviners, on the other hand, are seen to control vengeance sorcery; and, of male diviners, foreign ones and the Muslims are by common consent usually deemed most powerful. There are no female Muslim diviners.

Of the diviners, a general contrast can be drawn between those who act as spirit mediums, conversing with their spirits, whom they summon through the shaking of their gourds, and the Muslim diviners, who give a 'reading' by interpreting passages in their books. In the more usual, Gisu, way the diviner sits inside his house near his divinatory shrine and summons his spirits by shaking his gourds. The spirits arrive, are greeted as visitors, invited in and, once in, enquire the reason for the summons. The diviner then converses with them over the rattling of his gourds. Some do this hidden by a partition, but the more skilled ventriloquists are able to localise the voices of the messenger spirits in the shrine, their voices usually thin, high-pitched and barely intelligible. In addition to this direct communication with the world of the ancestral spirits, diviners also read auguries, divined by sacrificing chickens and throwing shells.

During divinatory seances neither kind of diviner is expected to become possessed or to go into a trance. The diviner works through his superior and special sensitivity, his heightened sensuous powers. His power of speech allows him to converse with the unseen world; that of listening enables him to learn through the shrill voices of his spirits; that of seeing – the verb which the Gisu use of knowledge gained through direct experience, as opposed to that transmitted through speech – allows him to detect the sources of evil that surround a person in the configuration of shells scattered on the ground or passages from the Koran. For the sorcery seekers it is their ability to 'smell' which leads them to the hidden substance. However, each practitioner tends to develop his or her own personal style and techniques, and I did see one diviner go into a possession trance. This was a woman who, according to the day, divined either by Gisu or by Ganda means. The day I visited her was a Ganda day and, dressed in barkcloth with a leopard skin over her shoulder, she went convulsively into a state of possession. Once the spirits had settled in her she conversed with them in a state of trance. All this conversation was in Luganda, and was translated to us by a helper called in for the purpose. Coming out of the trance, as convulsively as she had gone in, she claimed ignorance of the content. A foreign element is not unusual, however, in Gisu divination. Apart from the Muslims who have already been mentioned, the spirits of the gourd diviners often speak in foreign languages, often Luganda (but also other Ugandan languages) or even on one occasion in something that certainly resembled Latin. That diviner claimed the gift of tongues.

This eclectic mixing of styles undoubtedly adds an exotic element to the sessions and adds to the prestige of the practitioner and the mystique of the process. The foreign elements also add elements of power and danger: the Gisu, like other peoples of the region, tend to attribute superior supernatural skills to distance. They may also be said to reflect the range of influences present in the modern situation in Bugisu. But it should not, for that reason, be assumed that they are 'untraditional', for the point about tradition in the way it takes shape in Gisu thought and practice is that what matters is not only what is handed on but how it is handed on. It is the principle of transmission which is at stake.

Divination, as has been said, forms part of a more general set of ideas about the ancestral transmission of powers and traditions. The Gisu postulate a continuity of 'spirit' seen as the source of life existing on a parallel plane to physical procreation. This is identified in the *cisimu*, the penumbra around the shadow of a person, and is inherited by a child from someone in his kindred who has recently died. The child is given this name. In a similar way the major traditions/powers of the Gisu are perpetuated through a process of recycling. These powers, known as *kimisambwa* (sing. *kumusambwa*), embrace all the important Gisu traditions, which are transmitted from generation to generation by 'catching' people with the characteristic affliction. Through ritual a person is both cured and further identified with the powers of that *kumusambwa*. These they exercise during life and transmit in the same way to their descendants after death. In a general way these powers are associated with the *basambwa*, ancestral spirits, those dead who are no longer remembered as distinct personalities by the living, but are incorporeal 'like the air'. The ancestral ghosts (*bamakombe*) on the other hand are those dead who are still remembered, and their attributes suggest a far more ambivalent relationship between living and dead. Their interventions in the life of their descendants always bode ill and they must be placated to avoid further ill-effects. By contrast, the afflictions sent by the *basambwa*, though they cause illness, are a sign of empowerment, and allow the negative symptom to be turned into a positive attribute.

The powers associated with a person's ancestry are distinctive to it but some are extremely widespread. Divination together with circumcision and the power to circumcise is regarded as originating with the founding ancestors of Gisu tradition. Thus it is associated with Masaba, the founding ancestor of the Bagisu or Bamasaba, or with Nabalwa, the Sebei woman to whom myth attributes the introduction of circumcision. Through their common ancestry all Gisu transmit the power of circumcision, and likewise, with divination, practically everyone has it in their kindred and is liable to be 'caught' by the power. The characteristic sign of affliction in this case is a 'running madness', as it is often described, a derangement where the person runs and roams widely, without heed of his surroundings or caution for himself. At this stage it is indistinguishable from manias which do not respond to divinatory cure and initiation. Alternatively, *bufumu* may strike a person with wasting disease, usually accompanied by the death of children or barrenness. Again the severity of the illness is diagnostic of *bufumu*. This is a powerful ancestral power – one which can kill those without the strength to control it – and it tends to bring with it all the other powers in the kindred of the afflicted. Most commonly it is said 'to walk with' the power to become a circumciser, another powerful *kumusambwa*, whose diagnostic signs are similar to those of *bufumu*. Divination therefore always implies a multiple empowerment, and the shrines set up in the curative process in the courtyard of the diviner's house usually indicate a range of powers. This allows for the easy and regular accretion of new and foreign elements, integrating them with the fundamental process of transmission of power through kinship and ancestry. What remains unaltered is the principle of transmission, not what is transmitted, which is subject to constant mutation as the powers are brought into different relationships with each other in time and space. Tradition, understood in this sense, is open and malleable, not static and closed.

Consistent with this principle, the names of the specific powers that come with divination (*bufumu*) vary from area-to-area. In the central areas it is commonly said that three came together: Maina, Nambwa and Naxalondo, or, alternatively, Mukoya, Nambwa and Naxalondo. The first, Maina or Mukoya, generally indicates the empowering spirit which inspires the diviner, while the other names are those of the voices which speak to him during the seances. Indeed, Naxalondo has become the word used for the radio. But it must be stressed that there is little uniformity here, nor is there any in the genealogical relationships among the spirits which the diviners often proffer as a way of explaining the relationships among their powers.

Nevertheless, the foreign attributes of many diviners may also be seen to underline their social marginality. The prominence of Muslims, and of women who hold no other political or ritual office, is also relevant here. Interestingly, in the context of Lewis's (1966; 1971) theory as to the relationship between spirit possession and social deprivation, women diviners often appeared notably successful as women, and in this they contrasted with many male diviners. Despite the fact that the original possession had often manifested itself in the loss of children, depressive illness or madness, women practitioners were usually married, with children and even grandchildren. One man I spoke to put this down to the nature of the original possession, with men subject to the stronger forms of the illness which were more resistant to curing, though which, once controlled, implied greater power. Foreign experience, as mentioned earlier, also carried the implications of greater power. An example here is Tageti, a man in his late forties who made a living, though not a very prosperous one, from his divining skills. Though he had been born in Bugisu he had spent most of his childhood and adolescence in Kenya with his mother after she had divorced her husband. This experience was indeed written on his face, which bore scarifications, testament to his time among the Babukusu, and to the loss of his four lower incisors, extracted during the time he lived among the Luo. Yet, Tageti explained, he had returned to Bugisu to be circumcised and it was in that year, 1934, that he had been caught by both the power to circumcise and that of divination. His mania lasted a long time and he ran wildly, on many occasions risking death in his delirium. Nor, he claimed, would his spirits allow him to marry. Nevertheless, in this case, his divinatory spirits were all Gisu.

To conclude this section, Gisu diviners may be described in terms which have become familiar: in their centrality to religious belief, in their access to superior sources of knowledge and in the panoply of powers they claimed to counteract sorcery. The questions which follow are: why were there no renowned healers? Why didn't they gain a following and assert a public role? Why didn't their knowledge translate itself into social power? Here I must reiterate that Gisu diviners tended to be insignificant both personally and politically. Despite the extent of the powers they claimed, and while they could often be impressive in seances, they appeared to be very ordinary men and women outside that context. They possessed little charismatic power, still less the confidence of authority. Their marginal social attributes may be said to reinforce this position. Yet, in other contexts, it is this very marginality and the experience of great suffering which has been seen as the empowering condition, allowing an exceptional individual to articulate a vision which transcends the boundaries of the moral tradition to which he is heir. Clearly we must examine more closely the social content of divination in Bugisu in order to identify the social sources of the diviners' relative powerlessness.

The social context of divination

Initially we can consider how the Gisu approached diviners and what they expected from their consultations. Diviners were usually consulted only at times of acute personal crisis. They were not consulted for routine matters or to give advice more generally – for example, on rebuilding a house, the wisdom of undertaking a journey or the contraction of marriage. In most instances, therefore, they were a recourse of final resort when all other means had failed, part of a desperate search to locate the source or sources of misfortune. Here, one might hazard that people were in a highly suggestible state and more open than at other times to divinatory prognosis. While this is undoubtedly the case it is also true that people were not that open, since diviners still had to meet the test of credibility and it was a hard one.

The divinatory process usually divided into two distinct phases. The first was diagnosis, and a number of different diviners were often consulted, some of whom might live relatively near but others far away. People demanded at this stage – as they did throughout – a spiritual revelation, a diviner whom they could trust, who would 'tell them the truth and not just take their money for nothing'. Distant diviners were usually considered the most reliable, since their pronouncements were unlikely to be influenced by knowledge gained by means other than their voices, that is, not by local gossip. Further, people counselled each other prior to such consultations on the necessity of avoiding giving away too much information. They were unimpressed by those diviners who used their techniques as a way of eliciting information, running through one causative agent after another as a way of assessing probability in the reactions of their clients. They were most impressed, as any might be, by diviners who demonstrated some real insight into their affairs, an insight which could be attributed only to their powers or their voices. This was particularly the case on the occasion of a first consultation, where the powers of the diviner were being put to the test. A first session with a Muslim diviner may be taken as an illustration here:

> Charles, a schoolboy in his mid-teens, was suffering from a skin complaint sufficiently disfiguring to make him reluctant to attend school. He had tried various Western clinics in the area without success and was finally recommended to a local Muslim diviner. He went accompanied by his elder brother and myself to see Juma, who operated from his shop. The session began with Juma taking off his shoes and unrolling his prayer mat in a corner of the shop. Sitting cross-legged on it and holding the Koran, he began opening it at random, every now and then indicating that he had reached a significant passage. After some minutes he put the Koran aside and wrote out about five lines of what appeared to be Arabic script followed by two lines of numerals. Then he began on the diagnosis. First, he opined that the illness had been sent by the ancestral powers, a judgement he supported by referring to the writing on the page and again by opening the Koran. Charles and his brother made no response. Moving on, he suggested that it was the ancestral ghosts and asked Charles if he ever dreamt of the ghosts. That would disturb his mind and prevent him from concentrating on his studies. Charles denied it and went on to deny the next suggestion that maybe his joints sometimes felt weak – again, symptomatic of an attack by the ghosts. Well then, Juma hazarded, perhaps he had been bewitched? In that event, the book indicated, it would be someone related to him as 'mother', and at this point he ran through a number of common Gisu women's names. Charles refused them all. While the brothers waited as Juma ran through a list of remedies he might try if they returned, the session was evidently not felt to have been a success, and they paid their 3s. consultation fee and left.

In many ways this is quite typical of sessions which end as they began, indeterminate as to causal agent and to the procedure to be followed. A range of options, often, as in this case, running the gamut of the common sources of malignancy, are put to the client, who is left free to reject or accept them. Again, as in this case, people have their own very definite ideas about the likely source of the trouble, whether it was affecting themselves or a kinsperson too ill to come to consult on his or her own account. The boys' suspicions in this case were of witchcraft, and later, when discussing the session, Charles admitted that one of the names suggested had been possible. But, he said, he was not going to tell Juma. He wanted Juma to tell him. Thus, despite the emphasis on spiritual revelation, as this process of diagnosis indicates, it was the client and not the diviner who decided the 'truth' of the pronouncements. The diagnosis had to meet the acid test of plausibility, usually by confirming suspicions already entertained by the enquirer.

Further, in order to be sure of the identity of a given witch, it was said to be essential to gain the same verdict from three diviners independently and thus preferably at some distance. Even for those prepared to bear the cost of such extensive divination, a unanimous verdict of this kind was not easy to get. It was a rare divinatory seance – and I attended many – where only one causal agent was identified. A sick person was more often seen as under attack from a multitude of different sources; from the ancestral ghosts and powers and from several witches, acting sometimes in concert and sometimes independently.

Thus diagnoses were not by their nature authoritative: diviners had no power to impose their views.[2] And this was true at all stages of consultation, though, at later stages of the divining process, when the clients had accepted an initial diagnosis and had come for cure or counteraction, diviners certainly had more influence over the definition of reality. But then 'reality' had its own independent measure in the recovery of the patient and here, faced with chronic sickness and death, the hopes of cure were subject to constant disappointment as the disease proved resistant to treatment. Further, at all times, diviners operated in the private sphere as specialists hired by individuals for individual purposes. And this again may be seen to pose severe limitations on the credibility of their pronouncements. For, even where the client or clients were convinced by a divinatory revelation, others were likely to keep their own counsel. But, in any event, the results of divinatory seances were largely kept private.

Diagnostic seances were invariably held in the home of the diviner, and while clients frequently sat in or overheard the seances of others as they waited their turn there was no public arena for consultation or for the announcement of divinatory diagnoses and decision. Occasionally diviners suggested a public means for the identification of a sorcerer or curser but it was hard to escape the impression that this was given more for my benefit – as a possibility in the diviner's repertoire which I as an anthropologist might be interested in – than anyone else's. In any event, such suggestions were greeted without enthusiasm and to my knowledge were never implemented. Divination thus became public – in the sense of availability to public knowledge and rumour – only at the counteraction stage, whether this was in various curative rituals, sorcery searching at the home of the afflicted or in counter-sorcery against a suspected witch. But in no cases was publicity seen as a necessary or desirable thing in itself. While people clearly recognised that threatening to go to a diviner to discover the identity of a thief, for example, was in some cases an effective way of ensuring the return of the stolen property, it rested on the belief that the practice of sorcery against thieves was potent in its own right.

Divination thus formed part of a purely private system of self-help. Not only were its procedures largely secret but, existing on the unofficial level, it provided in many ways a complete parallel system of action and counter action to that available through the courts or by a direct resort to self-help. For example, Tageti, the diviner mentioned earlier, modelled his procedures on those of the early system of colonial chieftainships. He sent his spirits out as *banalukoosi*, the word used of agents of the chief in colonial times who were used to bring in the accused or, in this case, their spirit shadows (*bisimu*). These he interrogated with his *banalukoosi*, delivering beatings at his request in order to elicit a confession. If the accused witch in such an instance refused to withdraw his powers, Tageti would draw out and capture his *cisimu*, something which he said would not kill the witch but simply weaken his motivation so that he would no longer have the energy or desire to pursue the vendetta. Divination thus can be said to exist at a *sub rosa* level, its procedures and powers all shrouded in secrecy.

Divination forms part of the arsenal of weapons available to individuals in a system of purely individual self-help. This gives a further angle on the social processes involved. Following a death, Gisu lineage groups do not mobilise in support of their members, and vengeance was thus rarely sought. Nor is any tally of deaths kept. Thus, in the normal run of events, deaths whether by direct killing or from witchcraft – which effectively is all other deaths – do not call up in people's minds any previous death or deaths among the kin of the individuals involved. When a person is seriously ill his kin usually attempt through divination to identify his enemies in the hope of either placating or counteracting the evil forces pitted against his life. Death, however, is usually held to be the end of the matter and, although rumours as to the culprit are aired, action is rarely believed to be taken against the supposed witch or witches. Significantly, the death of children is most likely to precipitate direct vengeance sorcery, as the act of witchcraft in this case is thought of as aimed directly at the parents rather than at the child. Where witchcraft causes the death of an adult, however, it is seen to emanate from the specific hatreds which he had aroused and thus is not considered necessarily to pose any further threat to his kin. The lack of conclusive proof is usually considered sufficient justification for not pursuing the matter.

The ambiguity of divination and the reluctance of the Gisu to link murder or indeed any deaths serially gives an immediate, atemporal dimension to all such events. They are not seen as part of an ongoing history, as a series or regularised flow of events such as is produced by the action and counteraction of feuding situations. The Gisu recognise only too well that, in the words of one of their proverbs, 'The thing which kills you comes from your past', but such an event can be known only *ex post facto*. Past events have little significance in themselves. The things which have present meaning are the things which live in the memories of others, in their feelings and, particularly, in their anger, and this is essentially unknowable. This is the vision to which divination attests. It brings together events which have occurred at different times into a single constellation and posits that the emotions they aroused are operative in the here and now.

These features – the privacy of consultation, the search for distant diviners, the way they were approached only at times of crisis and as agents for private counteraction or vengeance – go some way towards explaining why it was difficult for diviners to gain wide recognition or build up a regular clientele. Added to which are the difficulties of another order which relate to what might here be regarded as divinatory success. For divination may be seen to fail at a number of different levels: in the lack of credibility of a given practitioner, in a lack of unanimity among those consulted or in the multiplicity of causal agents evoked.

Credibility and divination

An argument to be proposed here is that scepticism is endemic to the system and, possibly, distinctive to it. Evans-Pritchard's (1937) account of Zande witchcraft and of the way in which scepticism is contained and accommodated within the system, supporting rather than challenging its basic premises, has been seminal to understanding how people the world over are constrained by the terms of their cultural beliefs. A point sometimes stressed in this context is that we all accept our traditions 'on trust', and secondary elaboration is just as much a feature of the stability of doctrines and beliefs in the West. Thus there has been a presumed universalism at the level of commonsense thought, as, for example, in Horton's treatment of the topic: 'For all the apparent up-to-datedness of the content of his world-view, the modern Western layman is rarely more 'open' or scientific in his outlook than is the traditional African villager' (Horton, 1967: 186). Presumably, by the same token, the assumption is that we are all equally quizzical in our attitudes to our social practices and beliefs.[3] It is this view which needs to be challenged, because there is a case to be made that both faith and scepticism are socially conditioned. And here we might wish to reverse the conventional view which, following Popper (1945), has tended to equate scepticism with the modern worldview. Far from seeing our world view as 'open', setting free the powers of reason and the critical faculties, it can just as plausibly be argued, following Young (1971), that the differentiation and specialisation of knowledge in the West breeds an exaggerated respect for 'authorities' and demands that much of what is to be counted as knowledge is so far removed from experience that it can *only* be taken on trust.[4] By contrast, it can be argued that systems of knowledge such as that embodied in the Gisu divination, their groundedness in common experience and understanding, their very 'concreteness', as Lévi-Strauss (1966) would put it, encourage a sceptical attitude in the way those of the modern West do not. Thus, at the level of everyday practice, it is possible that we do not find a growth of scepticism as societies have become more complex but in fact a decrease. We are faced not with 'credulous savages' but with gullible modern publics.

If we consider the contrasts between divination and clinical consultations in the West not in terms of the differences in the content of the beliefs or their 'rationality' but in terms of the power relationship involved, then the following points can be made. In the latter case the doctor claims extensive knowledge beyond the cognisance of the patient, who has little or no access to it: the doctor assesses the significance of the symptoms, gives a diagnosis and prescribes a remedy, or refers the patient to a hierarchy of specialists. Almost total credence is demanded of the patient: at no stage can he challenge the doctor's superior knowledge. The divinatory situation is essentially different in its power relationship. Here, as previously outlined, it is the client who is the arbiter of truth; it is a system where both clients and doctors share the same cultural idioms, the same assumptions about human nature and the causes of misfortune. The diviner claims superior faculties for detecting the active causal agents, not exclusive knowledge of those agencies in themselves. Further, he is unbacked by an institutionalised hierarchy; there is no professional association of diviners, no guild acting to legitimate his sources of specialist knowledge.

The power of the Western doctor to pronounce authoritatively on disease depends on his access to a body of esoteric knowledge. This specialisation of knowledge in the West carries the corollary that knowledge is essentially nongeneralisable from one context to the next and its character is such that it is both untested and in most cases untestable by reference to experience.[5] In a very real way we have in the normal course of events no way of assessing the truth of information given to us by the many authorities or media of modern life. Indeed, it is this removal of knowledge from the common sense, from experience, which has been identified by Goody and Watt as one of the most salient features of modern literate cultures. And, with this, there have been seen to go very definite changes in the nature of the reasoning with which we operate:

> The abstractness of the syllogism and of the Aristotelian categorisation of knowledge do not correspond very directly with common experience. The abstractness of the syllogism, for example, of its very nature disregards the individual's social experience and immediate personal context; and the compartmentalism of knowledge similarly restricts the kinds of connections which the individual can establish and ratify with the natural and social world. The essential way of thinking of the specialist in literate culture is fundamentally at odds with that of daily life and common experience.
>
> (Goody and Watt, 1968: 60)

Access to the ultimate grounds of knowledge may thus be seen as inherently limited in the West, both in so far as in its abstractness it is removed from ordinary experience and, additionally, in the way it is organised hierarchically and controlled by specialists. But this in turn depends on people's willingness when dealing with specialists to expand their sphere of credibility and suspend judgements made in normal interpersonal settings. In all this it contrasts with the situation in traditional societies, where knowledge is available and based on conventional understandings which are widely shared. The knowledge employed by Gisu diviners is exoteric; clients and diviners are using the same interpretive schemas. Belief, one may hazard, is subject to more severe limitations as people approach these situations with a very different mental attitude. Unlike Western medical practitioners, Gisu diviners are 'tested out' by normal interactive criteria to assess their credibility on an individual one-to-one basis. Even more telling are the tests that, Evans-Pritchard tells us, the Azande sometimes put their witch-doctors to, for example, hiding objects in a bowl of porridge and insisting that the witch-doctor prove his prowess by revealing this knowledge. Of course, even in traditional societies some knowledge may be held 'secret' and form the basis of claims to special power, but even where it is so we may expect a certain scepticism to flourish, a scepticism which is bred in a pragmatic orientation to life's problems which is grounded in experience. Past experience is then the prime guide to belief, and where claims are made that transcend it the attitude is likely as not to be sceptical.[6]

If one thinks about diviners as operating in the area between hope, the search for some certainty in the face of chronic uncertainty, and reality, the inevitable failures of any curative system in the face of disease and death, one may perhaps see the band of plausibility as relatively narrow in systems such as that of the Gisu. And while it is true that there are limits to scepticism, the system cannot be disproved, since its idioms reflect back upon one another; its procedures may be said to encourage a pragmatic or even cynical attitude to divination. In the comparable Western context of medical treatment this is to some extent held at bay by the professionalisation of knowledge, as has been discussed, and by the constant lure of new cures. Perhaps an analogue here is with the periodic rise (and fall) of witch cleansing cults, with their new magic and medicines, which equally fits a current medical aphorism, 'Treat as many patients as possible with the new remedies while they still have the power to heal' (Gilmour, 1977: 157).[7] Occasionally an exceptional individual or an exceptional situation may broaden the sphere of credibility, at least for a while, but diviners, in the main, must scratch for a living in the relatively narrow area between hope and reality.

Diviners and social marginality

The atemporality of divination, its fatalism and, above all, the way it is resorted to as part of an individual system of redress and counteraction help us to understand the relative social impotence of diviners. Divination is by its nature a particularising skill, and there is nothing in the Gisu tradition which allows it to rise above its private and particularising roots. It has limited space/time implications. In this area of dense and continuous settlement there are no discrete villages or hamlets within which diviners could assert a public role. Nor is divinatory power articulated to lineage organisation or to modern sources of political power. As hired magicians they hold no brief for a collective cause. Yet they are not deemed antisocial either. Despite the hydra-headedness of the powers they claim, their powers not only of cure but of counter-sorcery, I have never heard of a diviner being killed as a witch. This suggests again that they walk quite a narrow path binding their skills to the service of misfortune, a misfortune that might come to all, careful not to make an independent bid for power or to be seen as agents of gratuitous malice.

Interestingly, this was not the case with the rainmakers, whose power to make rain carried as a corollary the ability also to bring drought. Localised drought was often attributed to rainmakers selling their services for the purposes of private retribution. Rainmaker lineages in central and southern Bugisu were both highly localised and very small, something which they attributed to the vengeance local people often exacted upon them. Experience of a drought in 1969 gave me some insight into their vulnerability as local feeling in the area hardened against two local men whose mothers had originated from rainmaking families living further up the mountains. Only the sudden breaking of the drought pre-empted a public trial and possible execution of the pair.

It is possible that diviners in the past also enjoyed a more ambivalent reputation. In the early years of the century both Purvis (1909) and Perryman (1937) wrote of the great power of sorcerers or medicine men and suggested that magic power was an important aspect of leadership in the defensive stands taken by Gisu villages against the punitive expeditions of early colonial rule. Yet it could be that Perryman has to some extent conflated the role of sorcerer with that of diviner, for, while stressing their potential power, he goes on to say that 'most of them were very poor men: they seemed content with the power they wielded and practised magic for its own sake and for small reward' (ibid.: 15). It is likely, therefore, that we are dealing with a persistent pattern in Gisu society.

Certainly it would be fair to say that, in the late 1960s, the Gisu had little in the way of a prophetic tradition. There were no stories of early seers who had predicted events at the eve of colonial rule. Nor since then has Bugisu seen the rise of any great millenarian-type movements or been subject to the ephemeral promise of witch cleansing cults. In the 1960s not witch cleansing cults but vigilante groups developed to counter increased fears of violence by the direct expedient of killing witches and thieves. In this process no diviners were consulted, nor was any appeal made to spiritual leaders. It is true that in the 1950s and early 1960s the nativistic cult of *Dini ya Misambwa* spread in from Babukusu in neighbouring Kenya, but it seems never to have gained any great following nor to have had great social impact. Nor was there, at the time I am talking about, any great upsurge of Christianity, in the form of conversion either to the established denominations or to new schismatic Churches. I heard of only one of these, *Dini ya Israeli*, whose New Testament Christianity was combined with Old Testament ritual, and whose influence was confined to a small congregation in Manjiya. In all this the Gisu contrasted quite markedly with their culturally similar neighbours, the Babukusu, living just on the other side of the Kenya/Uganda divide (see Wolf, 1977). In previous publications I have sought to relate this to the distinctive political history of Bugisu and to the economic power the Gisu peasantry were able to assert through the development of their own co-operative union to market the valuable arabica coffee crop (Heald, 1986; 1998). To be brief, it can be argued that the political culture favoured direct and pragmatic political action. The cultural and existential aspects of Gisu divination in turn reinforced its political marginality.

Conclusion

In conclusion, a return may be made to the social role of divination. The recourse to divination implies a special focusing on the nature of disease. As has been outlined, the Gisu line of first attack is directed against the somatic features of the disease or injury, through both herbal remedies and magic. When a client approaches a diviner, however, we may say that the locus of enquiry is altered, shifting from the body of the patient to the configuration of relationships in which he or she is involved. This seems a preferable formulation to that given by Horton (1967), who sees it as involving a jump from common sense to theory, a view which ignores the fact that the same 'theory' is involved at both stages and informs equally both the 'common sense' of daily living and that of the diviner's seance. This shift from the somatic to the social, from the visible to the invisible, gives a radically different model for understanding illness and misfortune. With 'disease' no longer manifested solely in the body of the patient the processes of cure and counteraction may also be located elsewhere.

This aspect of divination has led, in the main, to a positive evaluation of its social function. In Turner's work (1957; 1967; 1975) the diviner is presented as a clever social analyst, diagnosing and curing the ills of the social body at times of moral crisis. Through ritual purging and catharsis the physical body of the patient is restored to health along with the social body. Magic works or, at the very least, provides a clear course of action in the face of threatening chaos (Park, 1963; Jackson, 1978). The diviner cuts a swathe through the mistrust infecting a social group and, working within the idioms given by his culture, clarifies the situation, narrowing the issues down to point a decisive finger at the causative agent. The way is then clear for action and a reassertion of moral values and, even if this has a crueller side in, for example, the banishment or death of a suspected witch, the group is enabled to co-operate amongst itself once more.

But this optimistic vision cannot be accepted simply as it stands. If the diviner's role is to articulate the hidden and not so hidden enmities, stressing their harmful nature, it is not at all apparent that the end result is harmony and not further distrust. Further, given the fallibilities of the system – the lack of a positive identification of one agent, the presence of continuing misfortune, and so on – the end result of divination is likely not to narrow but to widen the sphere of suspicion. Clearly this might depend on the social context and on the nature of the groups involved. Here we might consider that where, as in Bugisu, the diagnostic process is essentially private and the diviner has no means of imposing his decision, the chances are that it feeds rather than resolves social tensions. When divination – as is often, perhaps even usually, the case – provides no clear course of action the suspicions entertained remain to be hidden in the heart until the next misfortune brings them back into play and into full consciousness once more. Divination here legitimises ill-will.[8]

Turner, who has perhaps done more than anyone else to articulate the positive vision of divination in his early book (1967), comes, in some of his later writing, to stress its more ambivalent facets. In 1975, in line with his vision of dialectical tension at the heart of society, he contrasts divination, which 'seeks to uncover the private malignancy that is infecting the public body', with revelation, which 'asserts the fundamental power and health of society and nature grasped integrally' (1975: 16). Here he sees divination as revealing a 'paranoid' style, plugged into a negative vision of social reality, the 'secret war of all against all' (ibid.: 25). Yet, while divination incorporates an implicit Ndembu theory of evil, this is countered in the positive image of human nature and relationships enacted in the great cathartic rituals of affliction, of which Chihamba is the type example. In this short article

I have not followed Turner in analysing divinatory seances at different phases in the social process, nor have I contrasted them with other forms of ritual action. I thus run the risk of stressing the negatives. Nevertheless, with these provisos I find it useful to follow Turner in considering the existential implications of such divinatory systems.

Gisu divination can be seen to have evolved into a very narrow niche whose parameters are bound, on the one hand, by the limits to belief, and on the other by a system of interpersonal vengeance. Exclusively concerned with the negative aspects of social relationships and with a system of counteraction which knows only its own terms – force against force, sorcery against sorcery – we may say that the socially marginal attributes of diviners represent a real social marginality. At best they are agents through which the individual can be reconciled with harshnesses imposed by his own destiny, of ancestral affliction; at worst they are agents of individual vengeance and retribution. This may be taken as more or less disqualifying them from articulating a positive, future-oriented vision on behalf of the community. Clearly it is not impossible, but the point to be made is that it is a huge jump from these humble practitioners, interpreting the present in terms of the past and trading evil with evil at an individual level, to prophets capable of formulating a positive social vision, a means of moving forward, on behalf of a wider moral or social community. The system, when tied to witchcraft counteraction, would seem difficult to turn round. In such situations it may indeed be a lot easier for prophets to arise and articulate their vision in very different terms. Perhaps the enthusiastic conversions to Christianity witnessed in many parts of East Africa during the past few decades may be seen in this context. The dualistic theology of Christianity allows for the differentiation of power into its good and evil aspects; for a world where witchcraft can be set aside and evil power laid down. Given the complexity of religious specialists in Africa and the frequent merging of roles, generalisations are difficult to make.[9] Nevertheless, this chapter suggests that practising diviners may frequently be the least qualified to spearhead such a process or to lead a visionary movement.

7

JOKING AND AVOIDANCE, HOSTILITY AND INCEST

An essay on Gisu moral categories

The subject of this chapter is the meaning of joking and avoidance patterns among the Gisu of Uganda. I aim to provide a new way of looking at a topic as old as academic anthropology, yet one which still presents itself as a 'puzzle'. Indeed, the very 'oddness' of African joking forms has led to the development of an interpretative literature around them and the critical parameters of kinship structure with which they are often associated. Radcliffe-Brown defined joking relationships in terms of their essential ambivalence. They are a 'peculiar combination of friendliness and antagonism' (1952: 91), a play upon enmity, which gives simultaneous expression to the common and divergent interests of parties to an alliance. He saw avoidance relationships as another means of achieving the same end, namely, of managing potentially difficult ties of alliance. The Gisu have both these relationship forms; indeed they might be said to have extreme versions of them. Avoidance between mother-in-law and son-in-law is virtually total, whilst joking between non-kin is marked by an exaggerated element of hostility.

It is not only these relationships that are odd but also the entire system of classificatory kinship. What, we might ask, is the point of all this specification of conduct? Why is appropriate human conduct cut up and distributed among different categories of relative in the way that it is? We might of course accept, with Radcliffe-Brown, that it works to regulate action and to resolve points of tension in the social structure, but to go further we need to inquire into what it is saying about the basic parameters of moral action, about the essential categories of social life and of human possibility.

I follow Schneider's (1968) lead in moving from a 'social' to a more 'cultural' level of analysis, from a dominating concern with 'structure' to one more concerned with 'sentiment'. The move is thus away from seeing classificatory kinship systems as echoing lineage structure and systems of marriage towards a more hermeneutic concern with the polarities of value which they enshrine. In this I must closely follow LeVine (1984), who has argued that behaviour such as mother-in-law avoidance is best seen as setting the parameters for moral discourse and behaviour. Rather than interpreting them as odd quirks of a system of classificatory kinship, they should be regarded as essential for establishing the moral verities it posits. 'Avoidance' as a moral injunction, then, should not be seen as restricted to one or two relationships in any system, to the extreme exemplars, but rather as providing a 'model for conventional moral behaviour' (LeVine 1984: 74) and thus part of a more general moral code. I want to extend this view to argue that these patterns provide not just a template for moral action but an implicit philosophy, a meta commentary on the nature of social life and its possibilities.

Therefore, I do not ask, as did Radcliffe-Brown, what particular problems are 'solved' by joking or avoidance for the organisation of social relations, nor do I ask, as did Freud, how they promote the psychic adjustment of individuals. Instead, I offer a hermeneutic account of joking and avoidance in Gisu society. What story are these formalised dramas of relationship telling? What, for example, do they tell us of the Gisu conception of relationships and of the problems posed by sexuality and violence?

The argument of the article is divided into three sections. In the first I offer a brief account of the basic principles that inform Gisu kinship classifications and behaviour.[1] I then turn to the joking relationship, *bukulo*, with its hostile forms of interaction. Finally I review some of the literature on joking in order to develop my own interpretation of joking and avoidance patterns.

The structuring of sentiment

Although Gisu lineage organisation is patrilineal, the stress on generation as a categorising principle tends to override distinctions in terms of lineality. Relationships are conceived to lie on a scale from familiarity to distance and respect. Familiarity is the privilege of those defined as equal in generational terms, but between proximate generations the relationship is dominated by 'respect', *lukoosi*, and between members of the opposite sex by the added sexual inhibition of *tsisoni*.

Lukoosi has a range of related meanings, all of which are relevant to understanding kinship behaviour. In the first place, *lukoosi* is respect, a respect which embraces not only the proper esteem rendered to persons but also a sense of the proper ordering of things, of customs and tradition. *Lukoosi* in this general sense is the fundamental principle upon which all orderly social relationships and conduct are based. A person 'with *lukoosi*' is thus not only a courteous individual but also respectable, honest and law-abiding. At its most general level, *lukoosi* finds expression in the detailed rules of everyday etiquette. In a slightly more specific sense, *lukoosi* is mandatory among all kin, who must show proper respect for each other by observing due decorum. More specifically still, it is the guiding norm for relationships among people of proximate generations where it carries more forcefully the connotations of distance and formality. The behaviour prescribed between the generations is thus an explicit politeness which must be maintained equally by both sides. Thus a father must respect his son just as his son respects him. The *lukoosi* rules here tend to render formally unequal statuses egalitarian in everyday practice. Both seniors and juniors address each other, according to sex, as either *papa* (father) or *mayi* (mother).

Tsisoni occurs between the sexes and operates to intensify the restrictions imposed by *lukoosi*. The term can be translated as sexual restraint or shame. In relationships between people of opposite sex and proximate generations, where both *lukoosi* and *tsisoni* obtain, familiarity is severely restricted. Conversely, in relationships between people of the same sex and generation, where neither obtain, familiarity and intimacy become possible and there are no restrictions on physical proximity or touching, or on topics of conversation. However, the more general stipulation of *lukoosi* in relationships of all kinds continues to hold, and poses limitations on the types of behaviour thought suitable. Specifically it rules out any kind of joking or teasing, the only exception to this among consanguines being in the relationship between grandparents and grandchildren.

These rules of etiquette point to the emphasis, throughout the kinship system, on the distinctive and antipathetic interests of proximate generations, and on the corresponding identity of interests among people of the same generation. This is linked to a radical difference in their 'sexuality'. Kinship etiquette marks out two distinctive aspects of kinship linkage: that which might be called generative consanguinity and that of conjugal sexuality. The first, the relationship of parent and child, demands formality and respect and provides the model for all behaviour between people of adjacent generations, who are all seen to stand in relation of begetter to begotten. Moreover, the two generations are seen to 'beget' each other in a continuous cycle: fathers beget sons but these sons in turn will beget children of the same generation as the father. This goes along with the equation of the alternate generations of grandparent and grandchildren.[2] By contrast the second kind of kinship linkage, based upon conjugal sexuality, colours all relationships *within* the generation, with sisters to some extent being identified with wives. This becomes clear in the rules regulating marriage, the use of bridewealth and attitudes towards sexual offences, all of which operate to identify the different sexual prerogatives of the generations. For example, the rules which determine the use of bridewealth bind together not only brothers and sisters, with the brother using a portion of his sister's bridewealth to marry himself, but also patrilateral parallel cousins and all cross cousins. These cousins are addressed as 'siblings' and all have rights to a portion of a girl's bridewealth and to inherit each others' widows.[3] Proximate generations are clearly opposed in these respects, for while in a single generation marriage and consequent bridewealth redistribution forge close bonds of privilege among its members, who may refer to each other's wives as 'my wife', this is translated into restriction and restraint between the generations. As has been seen, sexual distance is absolute between people of the proximate generation and opposite sex, whether kin or married to kin, all of whom may be referred to as *basoni*.[4] With them, incest or adultery is regarded as 'polluting', and not just 'bad' because it 'spoils kinship', as is the case with such offences among members of the same generation. Indeed, the collective interest of men of the same generation in each other's wives precludes any compensation being levied for offences such as adultery since it is considered that the woman was paid for by the bridewealth of the generation of kinsmen as a whole. Furthermore, the bridewealth received from the marriage of a woman may not be used for the marriages of men of the proximate generation, nor, in normal circumstances, may such men inherit each other's widows.[5] Thus, while the junior generation inherits land and other forms of property from the senior generation, the lines which serve to demarcate the divergent interests of the two generations are drawn with respect to sexual roles and prerogatives.

This has special significance for affinal connections, which appear as exaggerations of those found within the sphere of consanguinity. The simplest way to represent this situation is to concentrate on how, within the latter sphere, the parameters of *lukoosi* and *tsisoni* effectively create four basic types of relationship: those of same sex and generation (B/B, Z/Z); those of same sex, different generation (F/S, M/D); those of different sex, same generation (B/Z); and those of different sex, different generation (F/D, M/S). Affinal relationships may be seen to modify these in two directions: towards greater intimacy and towards greater distance. Thus one can plot relationships according to the degree of *tsisoni* and *lukoosi*, from intimacy to distance, yielding a gradient which in same-sex relationships runs:

WB/ZH – B/B – F/S – WF/DH;
HZ/BW and CO-W/CO-W – Z/Z – M/D – HM/SW

and in cross-sex relationships runs:

H/W – B/Z – M/S and F/D – WM/DH and HF/SW

In each gradient, relationships among consanguineal kin occupy the middle ground and those with affinal kin are transformations or exaggerations of these relationships.[6] Thus the lack of formal restraint between brothers becomes the 'mutuality' between brothers-in-law which is seen to be based upon the successive use of the same cattle to marry a wife. They are the prototypical 'friends'. In the same way, the brother/sister relationship transforms into that of husband/wife. One may note here that the sister is clearly seen as proximate to 'wife', not only in so far as her cattle are used by her brother to marry but also because she stands as the symbolic wife in her brother's circumcision ritual.[7] In the opposite direction, the father/son relationship with its *lukoosi* component transforms into that of father-in-law/son-in-law, with its more formalised norms of respect, and the mother/son relationship, already marked by both *lukoosi* and *tsisoni*, transforms into that between mother-in-law and son-in-law, with its requirement of total distance. This emphasises the fact that the contrasts are most extreme in cross-sex relationships which act to define the limits of the system, with husband/wife standing at the opposite pole to wife's mother/daughter's husband. Sexuality and avoidance could nowhere be more clearly opposed, and the relationship with the mother-in-law can rightly be seen to attest to an almost phobic reaction to incest (understood in the broad sense of the sexually prohibited), as Stephens and D'Andrade (1962) have argued.[8]

The relationships between wife's mother and daughter's husband and between husband's father and son's wife are both characterised as *bumasaala*, whose essential connotation is one of sexual prohibition.[9] In the case of the father-in-law/daughter-in-law relationship the restrictions are of necessity lightened due to the fact that, with virilocal residence, the two live in close proximity. The relationship with the wife's mother thus stands as the prototype for all relationships in the *bumasaala* category. A man's avoidance of his mother-in-law combines both fear and respect. Men say both that they respect and honour their mothers-in-law because women are more fertile than men, and that they are afraid to see them in case they might find them beautiful. Indeed, the prohibitions focus on the fear of sexual contact, of touching or seeing one another naked. However, the notion of *bumasaala* extends beyond this to include all that is obscene. Terms of abuse are referred to as words of *bumasaala*, which are thought to have the power to harm irrespective of the relationship between people. Basically, however, *bumasaala* refers to what is sexually forbidden and the restrictions entailed are of such cardinal value that breach is felt to be an abomination.

The set of attitudes associated with *bumasaala* can be examined further by looking at the connotations of *lukoosi*, *tsisoni* and the word more generally used for shame, *kamanyanyu*. These terms have overlapping sets of association and reference. *Lukoosi*, described earlier, can be glossed in the present context as 'respect'. *Tsisoni*, while it too implies respect, is of a form best rendered as sexual reticence or inhibition. *Tsisoni* 'catches' you when sexual distance is breached. The effect experienced here is likened to that of shame, *kamanyanyu*. Yet shame provides only a partial gloss as it fails to capture both the strength and the range of this effect, which also implies fear. Thus *kamanyanyu* may catch a child when he is scolded, but equally it might catch an adult in a variety of different but dangerous situations. One man gave the following list of things which might inspire *kamanyanyu*: all situations where *tsisoni* is present, walking alone at night or sleeping alone in a house, seeing a snake or a wild animal, walking in a town or seeing a murdered and mutilated body. *Kamanyanyu* seems to apply to raw fear, a sense of the ominous; it is the type of fear which makes your skin crawl.[10] And *tsisoni* is the strongest fear of all. Felt on the skin, if you look directly at your mother-in-law *tsisoni* can catch your body all over. Fittingly perhaps, the punishment, as with most pollution, takes the form of a skin disease.

To return to the kinship context for these attitudes, we may note first that mother-in-law and son-in-law are asymmetric with respect to the basic polarities around which the Gisu have constructed their kinship universe, that is, of sex and generation. And running through all these classifications is the opposition between conjugal/sexual and generative/consanguineal linkage. Here, the patterned discriminations extend into the most private and intimate sphere of social life. A woman's maternal or procreative role is clearly separated from her conjugal, sexual one, with the intimate physical relationship a woman has with her husband, on the one hand, and her children, on the other, being separated by ritual restrictions (*kimisiro*). Thus, if a man becomes seriously ill or incontinent a wife cannot nurse him, for only a woman related as 'mother' can wash and clean his anus and genitals. In a like manner, a man may never touch or suck his wife's breasts for these 'belong to the children' and any injury here is an offence which pollutes the couple and requires ritual annulment and compensation. Thus the Gisu are offered two possible but mutually incompatible models of conduct towards the opposite sex. Following Douglas's (1966) line of argument we may see mother-in-law/son-in-law avoidance as falling at the point of intersection between the two categories; a point which, dramatised by taboo, in turn serves to epitomise the lines of division between them.

Further, a woman's fertility is largely credited to her mother who is said to have 'grown her' and to have protected her from the dangers of sorcery and other misfortune during her childhood. A girl is most vulnerable to malignant supernatural force during her first menstruation and this tends to be specified as the particular charge of the mother, the essential part of any safe rearing. When a girl marries, the debt to her mother is recognised in the gifts of clothes, hoes and other household utensils which she receives; items which fall outside the bridewealth proper and are not repayable on divorce. Yet, in a very real sense, the debt to the mother-in-law can never be repaid. She has no stake in the exchange of livestock which procure wives for the male members of the family, and Gisu marriage rules ensure that women are not directly reciprocated between families.[11]

I have set forth the major contrasts which place the behaviour towards the mother-in-law at one end of a spectrum of possible social behaviours. As has been described, the wife's mother/daughter's husband relationship is associated with fear, a fear which hinges on a sexual reticence so strong that it amounts to dread and imposes avoidance. But what then do we make of the joking relationship, *bukulo*, which, as I shall describe, freely makes play with the things of *bumasaala*, with the sexually obscene, with violence and hostile abuse?

The joking relationship – *bukulo*

Bukulo is a hereditary joking relationship which holds between members of different lineages, linking them as joking partners *bakulo* (sing. *umukulo*) to each other. In outline, the pattern conforms to that widely reported in Africa, but differs from those reported elsewhere in that joking partners are neither kin nor affines, nor are they linked by the performance of any mutual service such as in funeral or purificatory rites. Nor do they possess any other role in community or kinship affairs such as that of mediation in disputes. The relationship is thus one which is defined and has meaning solely in terms of the license given by 'joking', and this license is explained in terms of the prior hostility between linked lineage's. *Bukulo* is thus presented as a peace pact and all its symbolic forms build upon this notion with its dual correlates of amity and enmity.[12]

Gisu joking is extreme and often startling. Joking partners are licensed to revile, abuse and insult each other Further, it is stressed that *bukulo* exchanges are 'not play' (*xung'aa*) but 'abuse' (*xuxomana*), and thus distinguished from light hearted jesting or chaffing. In practice the most extreme forms of verbal abuse tend to occur only between those men who are contemporaries and partners (see below) and, in my experience, interactions are more restrained between those of opposite sex. However, in principle, such restraints may be set aside and any type of abuse is licensed.

Abuse may run from relatively innocuous remarks over personal appearance ('big head', 'shrivelled body', 'unkempt hair' and the like) to more direct accusations of witchcraft and the types of animal and sexual obscenities which would in other circumstances undoubtedly precipitate fighting. Indeed, all rude personal remarks tend to carry the implication of witchcraft since they play upon the kind of objectionable characteristics which can be taken as the mark of a witch. If witchcraft is imputed to the recipient of the abuse, however, it is equally imputed to the perpetrator since open abuse and the utterance of obscenities are seen as a form of cursing. This is not to say that witchcraft and *bukulo* are identified in any other ways, but simply to emphasise the abnormality of the behaviour; it is beyond the pale.

Added to this, while many such exchanges are taken in apparent good heart and often accompanied by considerable jocularity, they can also be 'played for real'. In such cases, for the unsuspecting observer, they may be indistinguishable from a real conflict. On one occasion, when travelling in an area unknown to both of us, my assistant and I were caught out in this way and I still vividly remember the panic of our reaction when the local man who had offered to act as our guide was suddenly subjected to a stream of vitriolic abuse from a man whose house we were passing. Under this provocation our guide remained silent for a few minutes and then began to respond with equal vehemence. My assistant, as apprehensive as myself, suggested that we make a run for it before finding ourselves witness to a brawl or worse. As we left, both men were shaking their sticks at each other. Before we had gone further than a hundred yards, however, our guide ran after us and, catching us up, explained that we had no need to fear as his assailant was only his *umukulo*. Reassured, we returned and, with our flight at least having introduced some leavening, the two men concluded their exchanges at the level of badinage.

The scene described above took place between men who were linked as joking partners, that is by a special partnership contracted between individuals on the basis of the *bukulo* relationship between their lineage segments. While it is said that this relationship may be formed between women it is generally contracted between men, either following the final mortuary ceremonies for the father of one of them or after their own circumcisions. The relationship is developed by the reciprocal 'snatching' – known by the special term, *xutubuta* of each other's property. These thefts begin with small items, such as pots or chickens, and progress to goods of higher value, the aim being to snatch a cow from each other. Such snatching is done strictly by turn, with one man initiating the exchange and then waiting until his partner retaliates by taking an item of equivalent value. The way is then open to snatching items of greater value, and so on, with the taking of cattle effectively ending the cycle of escalation. Any further snatching between the two is then said to begin anew with the taking of chickens. The 'negative reciprocity of abuse', as Richards (1937) called it, is here carried over to the expropriation of property.

This snatching, and the possibility of playing it for real, are important to an understanding of the particular elaboration of Gisu joking forms. For joking relationships are said to originate from peace pacts, and these were the main way in which feuds and enmities were concluded among neighbouring people in the past. Hatred is re-enacted in the omission of greetings on meeting, in the seriousness of the abuse and in the mock thefts. This symbolic theme is further developed in the rules associated with the snatching. For example, a man cannot snatch from his joking partner until he has provoked the latter into responding in like terms. Apprehensive as to what he might take, those in the partner's homestead usually attempt restraint for once he has successfully 'picked a quarrel', he may strike the object he wants and make off with it. Moreover, when livestock is taken, as is most usual, the animal must be slaughtered on the path on the way home: it cannot be taken alive into the snatcher's home where it could then be used for breeding. *Bukulo* is equated with destruction: with the taking of life and consequent enmity.

Snatching of this kind takes place at yearly or even longer intervals and Christmas has become a favoured time for it. The Gisu see this progressive snatching as a way for the two men to 'test' the strength of their relationship. The toleration of such thefts is seen to strengthen the 'friendship' between the two. Yet this bond is of *bukulo*, and not of friendship (*busaale*), from which it is held to be qualitatively different by virtue of both its enduring nature and the element of hostility. It is said that unlike friendship, *bukulo* cannot die since it does not depend on personal whim or the vagaries of individual affection, but is a relationship which is renewed with the same force in each succeeding generation. Further, the symbolic theme of violence and hostility sharply distinguishes *bukulo* from normal friendship. It is seen to be grounded in bitterness, *cilulu*, a term that carries the connotations of might and potency. The most bitter medicines to taste are those deemed most efficacious; the bitterest experiences are those which endure the longest. Like kinship, *bukulo* is a perpetual alliance, but its roots are seen to lie in enmity, in past bitterness which can never be forgotten.

Yet, while hatred is said to underlie the particular forms taken by the relationship, the pact equally implies peace and friendship. *Bakulo*, under pain of the destruction of their lines, may not take offence or respond with real antagonism. Nevertheless, hatred is an ever-present facet of the relationship and is said to rise once more to the surface – to be an emotive factor in the situation – at times of illness and death when joking partners are identified once more as 'killers'. Joking partners do not visit each other during illness for it is said that if they do, the sick person will die. Again like enemies, following a death, they practise total avoidance, neither meeting nor speaking. This is further elaborated in southern areas of Bugisu in beliefs that the ghosts of the *bakulo* 'snatch' the shadow soul of the dead person, keeping it until the final mortuary ceremonies are performed. Then, in some areas, the living *bakulo* attend to snatch the tail of the sacrificial ox and the shadow soul is released to join the ghosts of his own kin. This is the only mortuary ceremony attended by *bakulo* and the relationship among the living kinsmen must thereafter be remade and the hatred 'cut' once more. Such ceremonies are effective re-enactments of the original compact.

The peace treaty which created *bukulo* was marked by the killing of a dog. This graphically represents the ending of hostilities by symbolically striking at the very motives which provoked them. For the Gisu the dog epitomises anti-social troublemaking, *kamaya*. It has 'bad blood', is described as indiscriminate in all its habits and proclivities, whether sexual, aggressive or in eating, and is universally despised.

Emphatically, the Gisu do not see the dog as a friend to man but more as the enemy within the camp; the unsocialisable domestic animal inherently opposed to the discipline and conventions of the human social order. It thus represents the disregard for normal conventions which leads to trouble and ill will within the community, and its outcome, hatred, *cixonde*. The dog is also the only domesticated animal which is not eaten, and this prohibition extends to all animals which fall into the 'dog' class, a taxon which includes most of the wild carnivores, leopards and lions. All associations thus reinforce the idea that the dog is a hostile predator which is tolerated within human society for one purpose alone, as a guard animal, where its natural aggressiveness can be used to fend off the danger from human enemies. Dogs are frequently beaten, starved and fed 'medicines' in order to make them fiercer. The killing of a dog to cement a peace pact thus forcefully carries the idea of destroying 'disorder' and all its associated evils. Once the dog has been killed, the two parties may freely enter each other's houses, their hatred removed, transformed into a form of friendship, but not forgotten.

The meaning of joking relationships

Radcliffe-Brown's (1924; 1940; 1949) series of papers on joking relationships in Africa has generated a vast critical literature and dominated the terms of the discourse over since. His emphasis on their essential ambivalence, combining both friendship and antagonism, goodwill and hostility, has been incorporated into the majority of analyses, even where the authors have been otherwise critical of his approach (for example, Apthorpe, 1967; Beidelman, 1966; Douglas, 1968; Rigby, 1968; Sharman, 1969). By contrast, some more recent commentaries (Freedman, 1977; Howell, 1973; Kennedy, 1970; Stevens, 1978) have argued that war should play down the hostile element and concentrate on the goodwill. I propose to deal with this position first, because I believe that it fails to come to grips with the abusive joking patterns of Africa and also runs against a whole current of thought on the nature of the joke and the comic. Bergson (1921), Freud (1960) and Koestler (1964) have all seen hostility as an essential aspect of the comic. Thus, in dealing with relationships such as the Gisu *bukulo* one can argue that there is no paradox but instead a neat symmetry of form and content.

Of those who have argued that Radcliffe-Brown overstressed the hostile, disjunctive aspects of joking, Howell puts the matter in the most general terms, denying that the 'need to symbolise separation accounts for teasing relationships. On the contrary, in most cases teasing appears to *deny* distance and to symbolise potential closeness' (1973: 4). It flourishes in the 'safe area' of social relationships. Thus, *pace* Radcliffe-Brown, teasing does not act to reduce latent hostility but rather develops only where there is none. Alternative functions are then proposed for joking-cum-teasing: it is said to test and affirm social relationships and boundaries (Howell 1973), to symbolise exclusiveness (Stevens, 1978) or to be a marker of special affinal solidarity (Freedman, 1977).

This formulation does provide a possible gloss on teasing relationships that are found within the sphere of kinship in Bugisu. The teasing which occurs here is explicitly seen as reflecting real feelings of trust and friendship, and to be incompatible with any actual conflict or tension in the relationship. Reciprocal relationships between brothers-in-law and between men who have named sisters, or between both men and women whose children have married, are seen as ideal foundations for the development of life-long friendships which can, and frequently do, outlast the marriages upon which they are based. These relationships are critical for developing the network of ties a man needs to facilitate the social round, and to provide for mutual support and economic help. Yet, although amicability is built into the terms of such relationships, the onus is upon individuals to cement them over time. It is in this area of social relationships that teasing or jocular banter is considered appropriate.

Yet with joking between affines the normal rules of polite behaviour continue to hold; a man must be careful not to overstep the mark. Occasional banter is allowed rather than enjoined between them. Indeed, in such relationships a man has the right to take offence if he considers himself to be abused unnecessarily. For this reason the expected forms are mild, and make play with the nature of the relationship as, for example, when a man addresses his wife's brother as 'my wife'.[13] The mutedness of abuse here – as Howell clearly recognises – comes from the fact that joking or teasing is an extremely risky strategy in social interaction and one that is always open to misinterpretation. [14] Further, the interactive strategy employed here is clearly recognised by the participants. For the Gisu, a playful exchange of insults is considered admissible only where there is little possibility of real grievance. These teasing relationships flourish in a relatively narrow sector among kin and affines who are defined as equal yet removed structurally from the lines of direct economic competition. Thus grandparents and grandchildren may tease each other, making play with the ambiguity which relates them both as seniors/juniors and as members of a single generation, but it is not deemed possible, let alone suitable, among siblings because of the likelihood of dissension over the distribution of property. Since all relationships among kin and affines are bound up with the transmission of property through inheritance, bridewealth exchange or gift, joking among kin is always restricted in scope, and can in no sense be regarded as a strategy for overcoming conflict, whether potential or actual.

On this point I am in full agreement with Howell. For the Gisu, joking among kin is only possible in situations where direct conflict of interests is considered unlikely and, additionally, where the personal relationship is strong enough to 'take it'. Given this overt frame, the degree of license involved is related to the actual relationship and may be seen to 'mark, test and affirm it', as Howell argues (1973: 3). If, however, joking of this kind only flourishes in the 'safe area of social relationships', it is clearly not the case that the safety of such relationships is given *a priori*. Rather, where such joking occurs it attests to the constructive attempts of individuals to build up amicable relationships. It is a personal achievement. Further, such teasing modes as do occur are a relatively peripheral aspect of relationships which are primarily defined and recognised in other terms.

In all these respects they stand in sharp contrast with joking relationships such as *bukulo*, where the reigning symbolic forms are antagonistic and where no intimacy is expected between the partners. A theory whose key term is familiarity cannot help us to understand such forms. My point is not that different kinds of joking relationship can be distinguished (this has been done elsewhere, see Sharman, 1969; Apthorpe, 1967; Rigby, 1968), nor is it that there are discrete types which must have different explanations (Freedman, 1977). We need to recognise a spectrum of different forms, built from a combination of contrasting tendencies and symbolic devices, variously exploited. The theme of friendship accompanied by a play on sexuality and affinal connection is one (see especially Kuper, 1982b), the theme of hostility is another. Nevertheless, in recognising this diversity, we should avoid any temptation to construct a taxonomy. Approaches which develop an opposition between the parameters of friendship/conjunction and hostility/disjunction risk leading to just such a position. To my mind this misses exactly what was valuable in Radcliffe-Brown's contribution to the topic, which stressed the mixture of attitudes involved. Here it is important to emphasise yet again that in Bugisu even the joking that occurs within the sphere of kinship and affinity takes the form of insults which, however mild, highlight potential aggression.

Indeed from Bergson (1921) and Freud (1960) onwards, just such a mixture of attitudes has been seen to characterise the comic. Thus, while Radcliffe-Brown's coinage of the term 'joking relationship' to cover the aggressive joking forms of Africa has often been regarded as a misnomer, this criticism overlooks the fact that almost any 'joke' contains an element of hostility. Bergson writes that 'comedy can only begin at the point where our neighbour's personality ceases to affect us. It begins, in fact, with what might be called a growing callousness to social life' (1911: 134). The joke, then, depends on an act of distancing, a suppression of sympathy which, in Bergson's view, gives full play to the intelligence, to reason, to exploit the risible absurdities of life. Koestler too, in seeing wit as an essential mode of creativity, argues that it has an aggressive element. Its one indispensable ingredient is 'an impulse, however faint, of aggression or apprehension. It may be manifested in the guise of malice, derision, the veiled cruelty of condescension, or merely as an absence of sympathy with the victim of the joke – a "momentary anaesthesia of the heart", as Bergson put it' (1964: 52). It is the instinct which turns aside the sword even by using it.

To suggest 'teasing relationship' (Howell, 1973) or 'privileged familiarity' (Stevens, 1978) as a substitute for the term 'joking relationship' is thus largely to miss the point, just as it is inadequate to the simple descriptive task of characterising relationships such as the Gisu *bukulo*. As a first step, therefore, we return to Radcliffe-Brown's insight concerning the ambivalence evidenced in joking and to his discussion of the problem in the context of kin classifications and avoidance.

How then might we begin to interpret these relationships? We might start with the idea that kinship of the classificatory kind provides for a structuring of sentiment, allowing affective behaviour to be distributed between different classes of people in different ways. This distribution does not exist in reified abstraction but forms part of people's experience of their social world and its possibilities. Further, joking and avoidance may be looked upon as moral dramas of relationship, dramas which break up the complacency of everyday forms of interaction and, in so doing, open up a window on the possibility of relationship.

Let me return, in summary, to the major themes of Gisu kin classification and etiquette. First, all kinship relationships involve restraint, *lukoosi*. Second, this restraint is more stringent between those of adjacent generations, who stand in relationship of 'parents' and 'children', and more marked still between those of opposite sex. Third, this goes along with a rigid distinction between procreative and conjugal roles and the confinement of conjugal sexuality within each generation.

Fourth, affinal relationships are exaggerated versions of consanguineal ones: intimacy is more intimate and respect more compelling. In relationship to a man, a wife thus stands at the opposite extreme to her mother, and brothers-in-law are more 'familiar' than brothers. Brothers-in-law, men whose children have married and men whose wives are sisters may indulge in slight jesting with each other, but brothers never. In the opposite direction, the twin constraints of respect and sexual inhibition find their fullest expression in the absolute nature of *bumasaala* avoidance between a man and his mother-in-law.

Thus the mother-in-law is the focus for the most stringent restraint, and the relationship in effect epitomises the essence of kinship rules which all involve some form of restraint. By contrast, the joking relationship rides roughshod over the distinctions of kinship and marriage with which it is held incompatible. Furthermore, the joking relationship can be opposed to both 'ends' of the elaborate system of kinship behaviours. Thus to take the brother-in-law relationship as exemplifying the mutuality created by a link of conjugal sexuality, we may note that brothers-in-law, like *bakulo*, cement their relationship over time by increasing the scale of their reciprocities, but whereas brothers-in-law feast one another, *bakulo* engage in negative reciprocity, a sanctioned appropriation of goods which are destroyed or 'eaten' by one side alone. In the case of the mother-in-law, distance is dictated by respect and the asymmetric gift of life, whereas the joking relationship is associated with death and mutual destruction. A triangulated set of contrasts thus emerges: mutual gift of life; debt of life; mutual debt of death. If we add to this set the relationship between those in dispute, we have a set of behavioural options as follows: amity; avoidance motivated by respect; licence; avoidance motivated by enmity.

These manifest oppositions between kinship and non-kinship, restraint and license, and life and death, may be elaborated still further. Indeed, one of the challenges of interpretation here is precisely the range of themes, contrasts and polarities that it is possible to identify. In addition, both the avoidance and joking relationships involve reversal. In the case of *bumasaala*, a marriage in effect transfers a generation of people of the opposite sex from permitted sexual partner to a category which is absolutely forbidden. In the case of bukulo, a fight or war can conclude with a positive transformation of enmity into alliance, conceived in terms of enduring and absolute friendship.

At this point we may return to those analyses of joking which have taken their cue from Radcliffe-Brown, and put the emphasis on ambivalence and the theme of reversal. In so doing they have extended the interpretative framework by explaining the cosmological dimensions of the pattern. Beidelman (1966), for example, considered the problem in terms of transformations, regarding jokers as ambiguous, liminal figures. But if jokers are mediators we have then to pose the question of what they mediate between. What are the relevant boundaries of the social universe? How indeed should the social universe be conceived?

In fairly orthodox terms one can see the social universe in terms of sectors of sociability, the gradual phasing out of moral responsibility with social distance, as Evans-Pritchard (1940) has explained for the Nuer, and Sahlins (1972) for 'tribal' societies in general. Kinship at the core may then be contrasted with enmity on the periphery. Thus, we might see both mothers-in-law and joking partners as intercalary figures, points of contact between solidary kin and hostile outsiders. But neither of these polarities is particularly well-developed in Bugisu: kin are neither solidary nor are outsiders necessarily hostile. In part this arises from the fact that the kinship universe is virtually all-encompassing. At the interactive level all are kin, either by consanguinity or by affinity. Parochial marriage patterns and the wide extension of kinship terms ensure that everyone is effectively related, by one tie or another. In any event, everyone is addressed by kinship terms. And, working outwards from the self, relations with distant kin or neighbours with whom only a remote connection can be traced are characterised by a dilution of kinship conduct. Taboos fade out, incest ceases to become meaningful, obligations dissolve rather than abruptly ceasing. And, at some point along this line, kin become marriageable once more. In fact this is what happens, with Gisu marrying distant kin, and marriage being not so much the way kinship is created as the way it is renewed.

Joking partners alone stand outside this normal schema of sociability. In effect they are the only 'non-kin' in the Gisu social world, the only people not linked by the bonds of sexuality. Thus, while one could see joking relationships as existing at the point of divide, mediating between a world of kin and a world of non-kin, this is not altogether convincing. As we have seen the relationship is made, not given. Besides, there is a more interesting line of interpretation. That is, we can also see the social universe in more existential terms, and the relationships of joking and avoidance as then representing contrasting tendencies in everyday life. The emphasis is then placed not so much on ambiguity and mediation as on the role of reversals in social life.

Analysing the reversals found in carnivals, Abrahams and Bauman (1978) have written that we should understand these not as literally involving 'the antithesis of behaviour at other times' but as giving expression to the disorder present, if disapproved of, in normal daily life. This is clearly relevant for the Gisu. The neighbourhood is the sphere of the most embittered enmities where conflicts over land, women and breaches of norms are most evident and serious. Avoidance of overt and public strife is an ideal, just as physical avoidance is seen as the main strategy for peaceably dealing with an enemy, allowing time for tempers to cool. This ideal is frequently broken. Thus one could argue that joking gives expression not only to the hostility present at the edge of the kinship universe, but also to the hostile sentiments present within the community itself.

Like kinship, *bukulo* is a perpetual alliance; unlike kinship it is based on the recognition of violence, on the toleration of the intolerable. To return to the symbolism of dog killing, one could say that *bukulo*, like the dog, represents the invasion of disorder and anarchy into, and its subsequent containment within, the sphere of order and etiquette. This is reminiscent of Douglas's (1968) commentary on the subversive nature of the joke with its juxtaposition of control and non-control. On one level, joking partners represent the reversal of the normal moral order and freely indulge in the forbidden words of *bumasaala*, obscenity and insult. Yet, on another level, the very possibility of such reversal points to the essential relativity of human social convention and the creativity of social experience. Pollution can be contained and enmity transformed into friendship; men can not only come to terms with their bitterest experiences but also do so in a way that creates positive social value. In the pool of human experience, the joker, like the trickster, can transform all things, making mockery of the most deeply held canons of propriety and generating value from the apparently valueless.

This, broadly, is Douglas's view. She argues that 'by the path of ritual joking these African cultures too have reached a philosophy of the absurd' and they have done so 'by revealing the arbitrary, provisional nature of the very categories of thought, by lifting their pressure for a moment and suggesting other ways of structuring reality' (1968: 374). In a similar vein, Handelman (1982) argues for the reflexive potentialities of 'play', with its power to take apart the 'clockworks of reality'. Despite the appealing nature of these formulations, however, I do not see the significance of Gisu joking patterns as lying here. It does not seem to me that these formalised encounters are creative and liberating. In any case, I think the message may well be more straightforward. For if it is possible to regard *bukulo* behaviour as a reversal of normal ideal sociability, it is equally possible to see it as an extreme type of it. We might then see the relationship as representing neither mediation nor reversal, neither liminal nor lucid, but as giving yet another twist to the theme of restraint.

This view raises different interpretative possibilities. For example, if one emphasises reversal, then the joking relationship may be said to give notice of the 'hidden' dimension, the underside of social experience; human nature perhaps set against the repressive forces of the social order. This tends to imply a cathartic model of process; with emotion being channelled and possibly transmuted, as was posited by Radcliffe-Brown's theory. This would also be consistent with a Freudian perspective. Alternatively, if one sees joking as an extreme type of permissible relationship, one end of the spectrum of possibility, then we might say that though it appears as license, in fact, like other relationships, it embodies its own given mode of restraint. *Bukulo*, as the Gisu say, is a bitter thing.

To expand on this idea, *bukulo* involves the systematic turning of the other cheek. Violence on one side is met with restraint and even generosity on the other, and natural retaliatory impulses are suppressed. The following text illustrates this point well.

> When they first started *bukulo* my grandfather went to snatch a bunch of bananas in the plantation of his partner. He struck that bunch so that it shattered completely and each banana fell to the ground. Then he went and struck down another bunch. After that he slashed the stem of the trees, felled them and went away. When the owner discovered this damage he asked angrily who had come to spoil his plantation. Neighbours told him that it was his joking partner who had scattered his bananas on the ground. So he went to his joking partner and said 'You have spoilt my bananas but as it is you who have struck them down then you may eat them'. This act strengthened *bukulo*. Then, on another occasion, he ran to his joking partner's and caught hold of a cow; he hit it, snatched it and killed it. He even ate it but his partner did not pursue him as a thief. And so *bukulo* continued from strength to strength, and it does so in the same way today.

Conclusion

I have argued that the structuring of kinship contains an implicit philosophy of being in so far as it patterns experience in terms of the possibilities inherent in social relationships. The basis of the Gisu social order is seen to rest with *lukoosi*, a restraint which is epitomised in the person of the mother-in-law who is revered by avoidance. With her there can be no social contact. *Bakulo*, on the other hand, may revile each other with impunity. With them, all and any contact seems possible. However, rather than either ambiguity or reversal being the main theme, I argue that the keynote is again restraint. The joking relationship may then be seen as a fixed point in the 'normal' constellation of social relationships. The play upon form which Douglas sees as the essence of the 'joke' is here turned back upon itself to constitute a mode of interaction, a class of relationship in its own right. Thus, it is not a fake form but a real form of social interaction. And, like others, it may also be seen to encode its own drama of renunciation, a ritualised form of self-abnegation. License is possible only because one has forsworn vengeance. Mother-in-law avoidance and *bukulo* may then be said to encode contrasting dramas of renunciation; of love and sexuality in the one instance and of hatred and warfare in the other; *eros* and *thanatos*.

My argument that it is restraint and denial which are being dramatised in both these relationships calls for a final comment on how far their forms answer to the particular dilemmas of Gisu society. As I have seen it, they objectify the basic 'problem' of order in social life, perhaps in a form which is more akin to a parable than it is to a direct moral lesson. Nevertheless, they stress the importance of restraint, a restraint which is centred upon the self, and which, in the absence of both segmentary loyalties and strong patterns of authority, exists as the only force for consensual social living. The extreme forms that both joking and avoidance take among the Gisu may thus be set against their equally dominant egalitarian ethos. The importance of control gains further force when considering the constituent powers of the personality. In particular the defining power of the male person is seen in terms of a capacity for anger, an anger which leads to hatred and is thus inevitably disruptive of social life. This capacity for anger gives added poignancy to the dilemmas of control, a control which is centred more upon the self than upon others.

8

THE POWER OF SEX

Reflections on the Caldwells' 'African sexuality' thesis

The boldness of the contrast made by J.C. Caldwell and his collaborators between an Eurasian and an African sexual system has provided
the most influential point of departure for recent discussions (both
published and unpublished) of sexuality in Africa, particularly those
set, as the Caldwells' is, in the context of the debates around AIDS.
However, to an anthropologist, their proposed model of an African
sexual system is misleading. As they point out, there has been relatively little anthropological literature specifically devoted to sexuality
and information thus has to be gleaned from works largely devoted to
other issues, for example, kinship and ritual. Given this, it is perhaps
inevitable that demographers and anthropologists will draw different
conclusions, conclusions that relate to their differing interests and
specific knowledges of African societies. The Caldwells' aim is to
construct a model of African society which is capable of generating
ideas about the nature of sexual behaviour and thus explaining population and fertility patterns as well as those germane to the spread of
AIDS. By contrast, my concern is with the values and morality
surrounding sexuality, and then, specifically in East Africa rather than
West Africa, where most of their research has been concentrated. The
essay is thus not intended as a comprehensive rebuttal of their work
but consists rather of a series of reflections, stimulated by reading their
papers, about the nature of sexuality in East Africa. Its purpose is to
highlight areas of disagreement and to both present and re-present
evidence from the ethnographic record in order to move towards more
satisfactory descriptive criteria with which to begin to think, as an
anthropologist, about sexual morality in Africa.

Africa's alternative civilisation: The Caldwells' thesis

John Caldwell together with his wife and various other collaborators have now produced a number of papers outlining their model of African sexuality (especially, 1987, 1989, 1991). In their 1989 paper, they aim to show that 'there is a distinct and internally coherent African system embracing sexuality, marriage, and much else' (1989: 187) which contrasts with what they refer to as the Eurasian system. The African system, as they see it, has evolved around lineage organisation with its emphasis on reproduction and descent. Despite the considerable variation they document in Africa, their case is that certain underlying themes relating to this run through the social systems we find. Thus, for example, the desire of men for descendants is dominant so that polygyny is common, if not universal, and divorce likewise. Indeed, they see the conjugal bond as emotionally weak, with both husband and wife retaining links to their natal lineages and sharing few mutual interests. The division of labour by gender, with spouses having different economic responsibilities, ensures that the conjugal household is not an entity even for economic purposes. Typically, they argue, wife and children form a unit whose interests are opposed to that of the husband/father.

All this has particular repercussions in the field of sexuality. Following Goody, they argue that the Eurasian system, with its emphasis on the inheritance of fixed resources, sought to control marriage and, in doing so, female sexual behaviour. Here, ideals of purity dominate so that they 'moved to centre stage in morality and theology' (1989: 192). By contrast, they assert that 'the evidence is that Africans neither placed aspects of sexual behaviour at the centre of their moral and social systems nor sanctified chastity' (ibid.). They, with a conscious play on Dumont, suggest that *Homo Ancestralis* might be a fitting tag for African social systems, as traditional belief was 'the religious form of a fixation on the continuation of the family line' (1987: 431). Further, 'virtue is more related to success in reproduction than to limiting profligacy' (1989: 188) and, as a consequence, sex is surrounded by little guilt. They tell us that most sub-Saharan African societies 'do not regard most sexual relations as sinful or as central to morality and religion, and, at the most, have fairly easily evaded prohibitions even on female premarital or extramarital sex' (1989: 222). The sexual relationship (despite the emphasis on reproduction) is thus presented as one which is not subject to moral control. In line with this, they aver that in Africa sex is 'a worldly activity like work or eating and drinking' (1989: 203) and is transacted in the same way.

That is, it is seen as a service which women give men in return for cash and support. It is because sex, whether inside or outside of marriage, is seen in such terms that it is difficult to recognise prostitution in Africa in the same way as in the West. Sex in Africa always has a potentially 'commercial' aspect so no sharp divide can be made between the prostitute and the 'respectable' woman.

Well, there are certain aspects of this picture that strike chords. Indeed, there can be no quarrel with their very thorough analysis of the patterns they discuss. My disagreement centres on the kinds of value implications highlighted in the brief synopsis of their theory which I have presented. Ultimately, their version of African sexuality turns out to be little different from the received variant; if the Caldwells use the term sexual networking, the message nevertheless is that *they* are permissive, if not promiscuous. In the Caldwells' view this is because lineage ideologies put the focus on reproduction which militates against any concern with chastity. This is a very narrow interpretation of sexual morality. There is another whole side to sexual morality in Africa which this account ignores but which is equally present in the anthropological literature.

A critique here might proceed by a simple listing of disputed areas of description: in the societies I know sexual behaviour is not so permissive, and so on. In fact, there have been some methodological critiques of the Caldwells which claim that they have been fairly cavalier with their source material, systematically underplaying the evidence of religious sanctions attached to sexual transgressions (Le Blanc et al., 1991; Chege, 1993; Ahlberg, 1994)[1]. Indeed, the patterns reported, with regard to premarital chastity, adultery and so on, are diverse enough for us to doubt whether there is any point at all in talking of an 'African sexuality'. But, while I too want to present counter-evidence, I want, as I indicated at the beginning, to counter in more general terms, so that we have more satisfactory descriptive criteria with which to begin to think about the values surrounding marriage and its morality. The Caldwells have thrown out a general challenge and this challenge should be answered.

One of the tasks for this chapter, then, is to attempt to redress the balance – indeed, to see African societies as preoccupied with sexual morality, a sexual morality that has to be seen, not surprisingly, in quite different terms from its Eurasian equivalent. A second, but related, aim is to reassess marriage. The lineage model which the Caldwells adopt denigrates the conjugal bond. The first is so dominant in their scheme that the second just about fails to exist, or rather, to be valued. But the one can only exist in relation to the other, and the intergenerational

bond is parasitic on the conjugal one; even patrilineages are perpetuated through women. This is a problem which all African systems
grapple with. Nor do they solve it in the same way: the ideologies are
various and contrasting. But, the reproductive role of women, their
status as both mother and wife, is a key element. In order to approach
this, I am going to argue that we need to understand something which
is overlooked in the Caldwells' account – that is, the power attributed
to coitus itself. My concern, therefore, is not with the economics or
micro-politics of marriage but with the values that relate explicitly to
sexuality.

Sexuality is something which is constituted differently in different
cultural orders and, if we are to begin to understand what often appear
to be paradoxes in the sexual norms of African societies, some contex-
tualising work is in order. Eurasian and African systems do appear to be
cut against the bias so that the two slide past one another. The
morality of one is not easily either recognised or grasped by the other.
Hence the Caldwells' problem in identifying sexual morality in Africa.
For them, apparently, it can only mean female chastity. They make
little therefore of the evidence of what might be regarded as the other
side of the licentiousness coin, that is, in the evidence of extreme reticence and restriction in the actual conduct of sexuality as it has been
reported for many of the traditional societies of East Africa. Not only is
sex emphatically not a topic for open discussion but, even in the
marital situation, the act of coitus may never be referred to directly.
Husband and wife can only indicate a desire for intercourse indirectly,
for example, by a woman offering food or a man asking for it. Even
among the Ugandan Ganda, alone in the literature described as having
an *ars erotica*, sexual intercourse could only be asked for in the 'politest
and vaguest of phrases' (Kisekka, 1973: 149). And we are told that
marital sex should only take place in the dark as it was immodest for
couples to see one another naked. Elsewhere in East Africa, the norms
surrounding sexual intercourse prescribe the particular positions to be
used, very often only one, and there are widespread taboos on touching
the partner's genitals. These kinds of restrictions call for some
comment, and not brushed aside as the Caldwells tend to do as further
evidence of an instrumental and prosaic attitude to coitus.

This is apparent throughout their writing, so that the practices that
they do report – menstrual, post-partum and terminal abstinence, for
example – are disregarded as moral injunctions. They are not seen to
restrict or impose undue limitations on the free rein of sexual
networking which they discern in Africa. Indeed, from the resolute
materialist perspective they adopt (which comes out in their choice of

Jack Goody as their anthropological theorist) moral rules which can be seen to have a pragmatic rationale as, for example, post-partum restrictions not only cease (apparently) to be regarded as essentially moral but are seen as a further impetus to male polygamy and/or sexual networking outside marriage. Thus, the very rules of restraint lead, in their view, to promiscuity. But this relies on looking at the system solely from the viewpoint of men, credited with a voracious sexual appetite, which again seems to have its roots as much in a Western model as in an African one. So, in spite of their aim to describe and establish an explicitly alternative African sexual morality, their whole thesis is underwritten by a pervasive Eurocentricity as to the nature of morality and of sexuality. It is also marked by the neglect of a female perspective which, even on the basis of the evidence they adduce, would give a very different view of the importance of sexual continence. Further, the picture they paint is incoherent. We are asked to believe in a *Homo ancestralis*, lineage man, who cares about reproduction but apparently has little reverence or respect for the sexual act itself.

Clearly, further exploration is needed of the values surrounding coitus and, as a mode of counter-generalising, I am going to propose that many – if not most – East African cultures can be dubbed 'respect cultures', and that this respect draws its power from that accorded to sexuality. There is a preoccupation with the control of sexuality so that the controls surrounding sex, and the self-control that one must exercise with regard to it, epitomise social and moral behaviour. Coitus is fraught with danger, circumscribed by taboo and subject to restrictions of a kind that are unknown in the West.

Lineage models

Let me start with the Caldwells' resuscitation of the lineage model. Anthropological debates of the 1960s were preoccupied with the status of lineage theory, with the accepted models inherited from Radcliffe-Brown and Evans-Pritchard coming under increasing scrutiny as the importance of alliance and cognatic ties were re-evaluated in relationship to lineage organisation. Lineal descent ceased to be regarded as the essential key to understanding African social organisation and kinship.[2] Where the Caldwells' use of the model has merit is in the recognition of a certain corporateness in marriage practices so that in many societies the payment of bridewealth from one lineage to another in exchange for wives, creates not just one marriage but a series of possible marriages. This has obvious relevance for the institution of the levirate and other forms of widow inheritance and it is also significant in the reckoning of what constitutes adultery. It may well be, as the Caldwells hypothesise (1991), that it gives rather greater sexual access to women; there is a degree of sharing of rights. For the Nuer, Gisu, Luo and a great many other East African peoples, it is not an 'offence' to commit adultery with a 'brother's wife'; at least no compensation can be demanded, as the woman is seen as married on behalf of the generation as a whole.[3] But to infer that this was 'normal', as they tend to do, is something else. It is likely that the husband did and does regard it as an infringement of his individual rights. For the Iteso of Kenya, 'As one informant put it, 'it isn't adultery; it isn't incest; it must be simple theft!" (Karp and Karp, 1973). The principle then seems to be rather the same as the inapplicability of payment blood compensation within the lineage, but that it could be a source of inter-personal friction in many cases is undoubted.[4] More obviously misleading, is the Caldwells' reduction of ancestor cults to lineality and consequently to seeing them as concerned solely with reproduc-tion. The important point is that agnatic (or indeed matrilineal) values cannot be regarded as any more than one element in these moral and social systems – and given very variable importance and recognition. To regard ancestor cults, as the Caldwells do, as exclu-sively concerned with lineage reproduction and continuity is just misguided, even at the level of modelling with which they are concerned. To see them as not primarily concerned with sexual morality is equally so.

This point is best illustrated with reference to an example, and I will now turn to my own work among the Gisu of Uganda.[5] In the Gisu religious system no cult is paid to particular ancestors, nor are they distinguished lineally. Rather, they postulate a recycling of life force (*bulamu*), so that the life force of the dead returns to a new-born child who is then named accordingly. Death and life are thus linked in a continual cycle but no special cult is paid to the ancestral namesakes. Nor is cult paid to other aspects of the dead as distinct personalities, except on an *ad hoc* basis when it is divined that they are causing harm, typically in the form of barrenness and death of children. Rather the dead fall into two main categories (not always clearly differentiated in practice); those of the shades of the recently dead who are still remem-bered as personalities by the living and the more distant, collective powers of the dead no longer so remembered. These latter are concerned not so much with the continuity of lines of patrilineal descent but are associated with the perpetuation of Gisu practice, both specific and general. In their specific form, they catch the living with characteristic illnesses which demand initiation into specific cult specialities. In their more general form, they are associated with the overall templates for correct social living, with the forces of the *kimisiro*, ritual prohibitions, which underwrite the whole Gisu moral order. These have little or nothing to do with lineality but everything, as I will detail, to do with sexuality.

Respect

The essential power of sex and the need for its control is evident, I would say, throughout East Africa. Most of these cultures conceive their social orders as rooted in respect; a respect which implies defer-ence, attention to proper decorum and, above all, self-restraint. A good person, we are told throughout this region, is one who has 'respect'. For the Gisu, this is expressed by the concept of *lukoosi* and given tangible form in the detailed rules of everyday etiquette. The principle of *lukoosi* applies in all relationships but more formalised rules of restraint hold between those of opposite gender and generation, the one difference operating to magnify the other. This principle reaches its most powerful form in the avoidance relationship (*busoni* or *bumasaala*) between mother-in-law and son-in-law. This is an absolute avoidance relationship; they may never speak or touch one another, ideally, they should never even see one another. This relationship encapsulates all the major principles of differentiation in social relationships; that is, gender, generation difference and affinal relationship.[6] I think it is not too strong to see it as a phobic response to incest, understood in the broad sense of the sexually prohibited, as suggested by Stephens and D'Andrade (1962). Its essence is sexual fear and shame and this is described in graphic terms. It is the kind of fear that makes your skin crawl. Understandably then, it is seen to impose total and utter distance and, just as the rules of *lukoosi* hold at all time and with all people, the fear of breaching this particular distance is ubiquitous. The Gisu tend to marry within the locality so that neighbours include numerous relatives in the *bumasaala* category who are feared and avoided. With a system of classificatory kinship, the category incorpo-rates for a man all the women whom his wife addresses as 'mother' and, to a lesser extent, he also shares the avoidance relations of his brothers and other kinsmen of the same generation. A man thus cannot go to a beer party, walk down a path or catch a bus, without checking that a 'mother-in-law' is not present. And, of course, the same goes for women since the restrictions are reciprocal.

These rules of *lukoosi*, underwritten by the ritual prohibitions of *kimisiro*, clearly problematise sexuality. The most flagrant breeches of the moral code lie here; in the touching/abusing/exposure of the body. All risk pollution and bring harm to both parties. Mother-in-law avoidance rules were in fact of such cardinal value that I never heard of a breach in all my four years in Bugisu. This was not the case with other avoidance relationships, for example that between father-in-law/daughter-in-law, which is less stringent due to them living in nearby houses. Here, though again rare, breaches did occur at the height of quarrels and disputes with for example a woman raising her voice to insult her father-in-law or threatened assaults by one or other of the parties. In the most extreme situations, one side might accuse the other of a deliberate exposure of the genitals. The transgressive acts here directly testified to the anger in the particular situation and in turn inflamed it, putting one or even both parties beyond the moral pale. The resulting pollution signified a total breakdown in the relationship and required purification and reconciliation. Before this occurred, such breaches were a focus for witchcraft and other accusations, the offender having shown a clear predisposition to witchcraft. Indeed, what is taboo and what is witchcraft meet at this point, just as uttering sexually-explicit words, all of which are regarded as obscene, is regarded as a form of cursing.

One important point about these restrictions is that they should not be seen as 'irrational taboos' whose strictures can be prevented by relatively simple acts of purification or protection. They clearly formed part of the moral subject, the person who 'knew how to act' and was a responsible and responsive member of society. In turn, such rules form part of a systematically developed moral code which, in a kinship-based society, focuses on incest and gives it a meaning which extends beyond the simple prohibition of sexual relationship. Incest rules, as generally understood, as the prohibition of sexual intercourse with specified categories of relative are thus only part of the picture. To understand the nature of the moralities with which we are dealing, we have to widen our concept of incest to give a more nuanced account of the basic form of the moral order. In the Gisu case, the fundamental opposition between the generations, creates a morality where rights and liberties allowable among members of a single generation are set against restraints and prohibitions between members of proximate generations.

A second point is that respect and incest rules of this kind impose severe restrictions on social, let alone sexual, networking. They also impose a general prohibition on open displays of sexuality itself. Modesty is deemed of utmost importance for both men and women;

sexuality is not a topic that can be openly talked about; nudity is regarded with abhorrence as a mark of witchcraft; and any breach of respect rules has the same implications. It is difficult to describe the force of these regulations since they are constitutive of all social relationships, and determine people's demeanour in all social interaction. They vary in rigour according to relationship – light joking and chaffing, even sexual innuendo, can be tolerated in some relationships, between grandparent and grandchild or brothers-in-law for example but not between brothers or husbands and wives. But the essential rules of respect hold throughout the sphere of kinship.

There is a further aspect to these restrictions which might help us to understand the particular rules that apply in the situation of marital coitus. As indicated above, the Gisu rules of kinship conduct are predicated on a radical opposition between adjacent generations. The lines which serve to demarcate the divergent interests of the two generations are drawn largely with respect to sexual roles and prerogatives. This is linked to a radical difference in their sexuality. Kinship etiquette marks out two distinctive aspects of kinship linkage, with what may be called 'generative consanguinity' opposed to that of 'conjugal sexuality'. The first, the relationship of begetter and begotten, demands formality and restraint. By contrast, the second kind of kinship linkage, based upon conjugal sexuality, colours all relationships within a single generation, with sisters in the Gisu system to some extent being identified with wives. And the opposition between conjugal/sexual and generative/consanguineal linkage, and the patterned discriminations which it entails, extends into the most intimate spheres of social life so that the particular prohibitions attendant on sexual intercourse draw their power from it. For example, a Gisu man is forbidden to fondle or to suck his wife's breasts because these are said to 'belong to the children'. The wife, in turn, may not touch her husband's genitals, and this has somewhat paradoxical implications from a western viewpoint because, when a man is seriously ill and incontinent, his wife cannot wash and clean him. Only someone related in the capacity of a 'mother' can undertake such care. Thus the Gisu are offered two possible but mutually incompatible models of conduct towards the opposite sex.

The kind of propriety in social life that these rules speak to is the mark of an adult; indiscrimination was seen as characteristic of children and animals while deliberate transgression was the sign of witchcraft. This is of importance in understanding the role of initiation ceremonies and the way they are seen to create adult personalities: as persons in proper control of themselves and their potentialities. In the majority of Bantu-speaking societies in Kenya, adulthood is acquired by men through undergoing the rituals of male circumcision and, in some, this is accompanied by clictoridectomy for women. Their explicit purpose is often proffered in terms of the need to instil respect, to make the individual ready to take on the burden of adulthood. Indeed, the recently circumcised often comment that now they 'know how to behave', said in a way that makes it clear that they derive considerable pride from this. Another – but related – value is that of self-mastery; evident in the degree of fortitude and stoicism that must be displayed during initiation, and reinforced by the teachings and tenor of the ritual. The Gisu man is deemed to learn how to experience anger and how, thereby, to control it.[7] In other societies, among the Meru and Kikuyu for example, the virtues of self control extended more explicitly to sexual restraint – and not only for women in these two societies, both of practise female clictoridectomy as well as male circumcision.[8]

Restrictions on sexuality on the part of both men and women were called for on many occasions. To take just one example here, for the Igembe clan of the Meru, Jane Chege writes that coitus was 'a central religious act, the medium for the reception of blessings or to seal a curse' (1993: 187). It was used to receive blessings and to cleanse impurity, both on an individual and community level. Thus, ritual sexual intercourse was mandatory at some times and abstention was equally prescribed at others, for example, following death when all members of a village had to abstain for up to two months. Further, sexual relations were regulated by an elaborate series of prohibitions, which determined not only permissible partners, places and times but, as among the Gisu, the details of the act of coitus itself. She writes, 'the sexual ethic was severely restrictive, imposing sanctions on pre-marital and extra-marital relationships, and requiring abstinence from both men and women following births and deaths' (ibid.: 190). She quotes Lambert, an early British administrator, that in Meru 'customary opportunities for intercourse are in fact reduced in native life to a rarity which the European would certainly find irksome' (Lambert 1912–18: 15; ibid.: 199).

And just as conjugal sexuality was subject to restriction in many East African societies, nor does it appear that premarital chastity was taken lightly. The record on this is extremely varied but, if one uses one of the same source books (Molnos, 1973) as the Caldwells, one can find not, as they claim, a general lack of value placed on virginity, but the opposite.[9] Prestige and value was set on the virgin bride. Extra bridewealth was paid, cattle slaughtered in her honour, and there was corresponding shame where this was not the case. Indeed, the practices of many of these peoples in the past imposed severe restrictions on premarital sexual relations, most often policed (not by parents since the respect rules largely outlawed any direct interference or indeed knowledge of their children's sexuality) but by the age group. For example, among the Meru, although circumcision gave the initiate the right to engage in coitus, the sexual behaviour of warriors was controlled.[10] It was believed that coitus sapped a youth's strength and he had to avoid women and girls. Junior warriors were segregated in barracks and their behaviour controlled by their seniors. Even for the senior warriors, coitus was allowed only between engaged couples and meetings always had to take place in the girl's home and, according to Chege, with the warrior accompanied by several of his age mates. Coitus in the bush was regarded as deeply polluting.

None of this necessarily restricts sexual access and behaviour; there is always a norms and behaviour issue, as the Caldwells point out. But in this context we need to consider the particular nature of the marriage system. The Gisu, although predominantly monogamous, had fairly unstable marriage patterns, especially in the early years of marriage and there was therefore a fair change-over of sexual partners, especially among the relatively young. I suppose that they could be regarded as near the permissive end of the East African spectrum. Even here, the idea of marriage as creating an enduring relationship was given recognition in the obligation of a woman to return to undergo the mourning rituals for her first husband. In other East African societies marriage was more clearly seen as an indissoluble alliance. In some, until very recently, there was effectively no divorce once a woman has borne children, for example, among the Luo and Kuria of Nyanza Province in Kenya,[11] and the virtue of faithfulness – at least on the part of women – is stressed. And it is sanctionable. Among the Luo, each birth is 'tested out' by an act of intercourse by husband and wife shortly after the birth of the baby, an act which it is believed will kill the child if its blood is not compatible (Parkin, 1973); and similar practices are reported elsewhere. We would have to infer either considerable disbelief or disregard on the part of women for the health of their children for this not to act as a deterrent to adultery. And while the rules do not always seem to bar male adultery, it raises the question of who exactly they were being adulterous with in societies with a young age of marriage for women? Elsewhere, male adultery also carried its own dangers. For example, for the Kenyan Gusii, LeVine writing in the 1950s, says that the belief that two men of the same clan sleeping with the same women would presage death if they visited the other while sick, together with the rules on intergenerational respect and those concerning the effects of female adultery, 'operated to keep the amount of adultery among the Gusii at what seems a low level' (1959: 973).

There is a limit to how far this quoting of examples is helpful to the debate: one instance from the ethnographic record can easily be countered by another. Yet, if it only reinforces the evidence as to the huge variability of sexual norms in Africa, it does serve a purpose when the issue is an overall – if, admittedly, hypothetical – model of sexuality for sub-Saharan Africa. As I indicated at the beginning, what the Caldwells' model really fails to do is to grasp the essential sacredness of sex in Africa. But, the centrality given to reproduction, its indivisibility from human purpose, gives sexuality in the cosmologies of which I am familiar, a cosmic power. Again, to quote Chege on the Meru, it was deemed 'the channel through which individual and community life was renewed and also the conduit for mystical good and ill. It was always a highly charged act, believed to pollute as well as capable of cleansing pollution. The same act thus contained both potential goodness and danger depending on the circumstances.' (Chege, 1993:186).

Metaphor of mixing

In order to understand how this power is conceived, I now want to explore some of the metaphors used for coitus and reproduction. One common metaphor used in East Africa is 'mixing'; a mixing which has both sociological and cosmological dimensions. In the first place, coitus and conception is associated with the mixing of 'bloods'; semen being generally referred to as 'white blood' while the 'red blood' of women is identified with that of menstruation. This is associated with a widely-held procreation belief that a child is formed through the mixing of these two bloods. In some cases, the white blood is seen to effectively fix the menstrual blood inside the woman and the specific powers given to the white versus the red blood do vary. However, in its general form, the belief has three main implications: first, that the child is formed jointly from the bodily substances of both husband and wife; second, that repeated intercourse is necessary for conception and for the growth of the foetus in the womb; and third, very frequently, the most fertile time of the month is identified with menstruation and the days immediately following it.

So far I have generalised for East Africa but in order to explore the power of this 'mixing' metaphor, I need to return briefly to my own material on the Gisu. In Bugisu it has wide ramifications, since it sets up a range of associations which link procreation to fermentation and these, in turn, to anger. Beer making and fermentation provides the key model here, both for gestation and also for the nature of the changes involved in turning 'boys' into 'men' during the circumcision rituals.[12] Indeed, fermentation exemplifies creative process, seen in terms of 'bubbling' mixtures. Just as the beer bubbles in the process of fermentation, so women bubble with children and men bubble with anger during initiation. Pregnancy is also seen as a time of emotional turbulence for a woman, again linked to the volatile mixing of substances in the womb. All these generative processes are also seen as indicative of the presence of the ancestors and also tie in with another important metaphor, that of 'spoiling'; the breaking of the physical integrity of the substance or person in order to release its generative potential. Thus millet must be 'spoilt' in order to ferment, a boy must submit his body to other men to be 'spoilt' at circumcision, and a woman, in turn, offers her body to her husband to be 'spoilt' by the rupturing of her hymen. Thus, for both men and women, being spoilt is identified with adulthood and future procreation.[13] But let me keep to the mixing metaphor because this gives us another insight into the significance of sexual continence, as just not 'pure' or 'impure', or a method of fixing blessings or curses, but to do with the particular way its power is conceived. In Bugisu, I think that there is no idea that coitus in itself was 'impure', only that 'wrong mixing' is. It is wrong mixing that makes sex dangerous both in itself and in relation to other things. Further to the south, among Kaguru, Bemba, Nyakyusa, Zulu among others, there is a dangerous polarity between sex/fire/cooking and wives are responsible for cleansing the act of conjugal coitus in order to avoid the dangerous conjunction of the powers of heat.[14] The Gisu powers of creation are not specifically associated with heat but, as I have detailed, with beer-brewing, fermentation and the situations of change with which they are associated. Thus, people must abstain while brewing beer otherwise it is said that the beer will become too strong/sour. People in the compound should also abstain while a boy is curing after circumcision, lest their activity delay his healing, causing his blood to flow, and so on.

At death, the bereaved spouse must also abstain but, unlike the examples cited above, this is not due to a presumed positive interaction. Rather, it is due to its opposite, to a state of impurity linked to death and linked to the spouse. Intercourse is used here by the living spouse to remove pollution and transfer its contagion. This is a dangerous act and widows and widowers are required to walk far from their houses to find an unwitting partner. If the two ever see each other again, it is believed that death will result. The act, however, finally frees the bereaved from the influence of the spouse's shade and allows a man to resume sexual relations with his other wife (if he has one) or a widow to be inherited by one of his kinsmen.

In the context of death, coitus is thus presented as a positive counter, neutralising its pollution. It is also used to counter death in other ways. At the time of mourning, for the three days of the wake after the funeral, kin sleep in and around the dead person's house. There is dancing and music, explicitly to 'cheer up' the bereaved, as a widow in particular is thought to be in acute danger from the dead man's shade which may cause her to commit suicide and follow him to the grave. This belief speaks to the power of the conjugal bond. Other practices speak of the power of sexuality itself for the time of the wake is also said to be one of licence, when people may 'mix' at will, relative with relative, without it causing any trouble.[15] Like many other ethnographers, I imagine, I cannot actually testify to this occurring but I have no reason to believe that it did not. There is a certain aptness in the symbolism whereby in this most liminal period of all following an interment all normal restrictions are set aside. It is also concordant with the rather defiant attitude the Gisu took towards death and with the dialectical play of oppositions with which they structure their social existence. This kind of transgressive behaviour following death was also the only occasion of its type. It was regarded in a significantly different light from the courting which may go on between unmarried men and women following other rituals, such as aggregation rites following circumcision. Normal rules of incest would still apply on such occasions.

Practices of the same general type are also found in nearby societies of the Luyia group but with characteristic differences due to their particular socio-cultural orders. Thus, for the Marachi it is not sex as such which is opposed to death but specifically conjugal intercourse. Marachi again use the 'mixing' metaphor, and the widow here must have conjugal intercourse with the heir together with his other wives to lift the impurity of death by this act of proper mixing. Yet, again, this is an odd act which runs starkly against the normal rules of marital propriety, as the husband should on this occasion make love to all his wives together on the same bed. Nevertheless, Whyte writes that conjugal intercourse is presented 'as the essence of order' and used to defeat the disorder of death (1990: 102). This raises another important theme which is the emphasis on ordered sexuality in East Africa, an order which is identified with the conjugal bond. Reproductive power is recognised as something which needs to be brought under social control; through initiation rituals which recognise the individual as sexually mature; through marriage which defines the proper sphere of sexuality and legitimises the offspring; and later, in many societies, by terminal abstinence on the part of the senior generation when they hand over their reproductive powers to their children. As Whyte makes clear for the Marachi, conjugal sexuality provides the principle of order in human existence, an order created jointly by husband and wife.

At this point, one can ask what such mourning rituals imply for the closeness of the conjugal bond. Among the Gisu, at death, the social world around the deceased is dissolved, as relatives sever their connec- tion with the dead person. For the majority of relatives, this occurs three days after the funeral when the first cleansing rites are performed. Close relatives must still refrain from normal life for three to four weeks, until the time when the rites that will allow them to work and resume normal activities are performed. The widow's period of mourning is however much more protracted; it is her tie with her husband which is the last to be dissolved. I think it is important to stress that this protracted mourning is not seen as a penance; it is not believed that spouse might have killed the dead person but is attributed to the strength of the bond and the consequent hold of the ghost, which is depicted as haunting the house, attempting to make the widow follow him to the grave.

Affection

With this in mind we can return to the Caldwells' stance on the emotional poverty of African marriages. How justified is their picture of an 'African sexuality' stripped of emotional considerations because it is claimed there is little in the way of a close affective bond between partners? The obvious problem here is: however, can one judge, except impressionistically? While a certain distance between spouses has often been reported by ethnographers, I find it hard to see African marriages in the societies I know best as any better or worse than ours. Some Gisu marriages, some Kuria ones, are successful and others less so. In both, failure is deplored and put down to the personality faults of one or other of the partners. In both, although not expressed in terms of an ideology of romantic love, close companionship is desired. And in both, despite radically different household structures, marriage is seen as an enduring commitment. Ideally, the wife is seen by the husband as a partner and loyal friend. This is possibly more evidently the case for the Gisu where the conjugal family is the basic family form. That is, all the virtues that supposedly reside in kinship (mutual aid, brotherly affection and so on) at both the ideological and practical levels here reside primarily with the spouse and then, of course, only for the

luckier individuals with successful marriages. Among the Gisu, relationships with lineage members are coloured by ambivalence, by the
suspicions which came from them being competitors for basic
resources. Even setting this aside, a Gisu man can never rely on a
brother as he can on a wife, whether this is in the joint effort involved
in cultivating the land and bringing up a family or more generally in
protecting his interests. Further, the attitude to the wife is extended to
brothers-in-law who are seen as prototypical friends. Thus, it is from
among his brothers-in-law that a man builds up his personal sphere of
male friendship; it is to them that he looks for mutual help and largely
with them that he makes important transactions, for example, land
purchases and sales.

In the Gisu case, then, we have a fairly clear division between
consanguinity and alliance, with the relationships created through
women (and thus through conjugal sexuality) within the generation
carrying the important affective bonds. It is relevant to note that the
Gisu do not have the avunculate in the sense that familiarity and
affection are not characteristic of the mother's brother/sister's son relationship. Thus, in the terms that I have used above, it is clearly
conjugal sexuality rather than generative consanguinity, whether
within the lineage or among other consanguines, which carries the
effective load.

Alliance and contract

Let me now return briefly to the mixing metaphor on which the
conjugal relationship is based and speculate a little more on some of its
potential implications. Men and women among the Gisu are seen to
mix each other's bloods to create a child which unifies them. Yet, for
this very reason, the sexual act is profoundly ambiguous – life-giving,
but also dangerous because of its infringement of the bodily integrity of
the person, with all the risk of witchcraft which that entails. All bodily
effluvia, including half-eaten food and the earth from one's footprints,
it is believed may be used in the practice of witchcraft. In the light of
this, we might say that sexual intercourse becomes the ultimate act of
trust; both partners risk their life to the other. In fact, in Bugisu this
potentiality was more or less totally subdued. Witchcraft believed to be
practised by spouses against each other was extremely rare.

But if the metaphor of 'mixing blood' serves as a model for alliance,
then it offers the possibility that it is more widely the model for
contractual relationships. I have in mind here, the other main kind of
contractual relationships in East Africa, 'blood brotherhood'. Since

Evans-Pritchard (1933) we have recognised the term as a misnomer. He argued that it had little to do with 'brotherhood' or consanguinity; rather, it should be seen as a magical covenant formed on the basis of an exchange of blood. It serves thus as a rival form of relatedness. And, it seems that in much of East Africa – particularly Uganda – its symbolism relates directly to marriage, making the partners symbolic 'spouses'. A paper by White (1994) supports this observation. She notes that in several Ugandan societies, it is the symbolism of coitus, of the sharing of bodily fluids, which pervades the rituals which create the relationship and which make it binding. Apart from the mixing of their blood, often taken from cuts in the arm, usually in or on food, to be shared by the two, in some societies the partners had to sleep together on the same mat, their legs entwined on the night they formed the relationship. The fact that the relationship was explicitly likened to marriage meant that a man and his wife could not make the relationship, for example, among the Nyoro because it was deemed that they had, in fact, already made it. In other societies, the Ganda for example, it was considered undesirable between married couples as it would effectively redouble the force of marriage, making it too strong. Among the Gisu, though its dominant use in the past was to create inter-tribal ties, the only contemporary case I came across was between a boy and girl who used it as a pledge to future marriage.

We might infer from this that in these societies marriage, based on the intermingling of bodily fluids, serves as the prototype for contractual relationships which are felt as absolutely binding. Blood friends very typically pledge enduring friendship and unequivocal help to each other; pledges which they may not renege on for fear of death. This ideal of friendship is a much stronger commitment than that owed, say, by brother to brother and, as I have indicated, may in some societies such as the Gisu, through the working of affinal ties – at one degree removed from the absolute terms of 'blood alliance' – be the basis for personal networks of friendships quite distinct from those formed on the basis of lineage or consanguinity.

In this chapter I have concentrated on the inherent values that seem to reside in sexuality in what can be thought of as 'traditional' rural life and culture, and then in a somewhat schematic and tentative way. In this I have followed the Caldwells whose models of both European and African sexuality are based they claim on past tendencies: they are pictures of a past projected into the present. Their thesis rests on the idea that the tendencies they have identified are so deeply rooted that they will go on reproducing themselves. In the African case, therefore, they consider that modern economic changes, mobility, the concentration of people in the urban centres, and so on, operate to open up more options and thus extend the sphere of sexual networking but this is a matter more of degree rather than of kind. It is this assumption which is open to doubt. They totally fail to comment on how current European sexual morality can be squared with the female chastity they claim as its central value. If the last thirty years have seen wholesale changes in 'our' morality, the same is equally likely to be true for Africa. Indeed, arguably, given the radical and disjunctive nature of the transformational processes in both colonial and post-colonial Africa, and the very rapidity with which many of the traditional sexual regulations and norms broke down in well-attested cases following early colonial contact, it is to change and not to continuity that we should be looking. But here we need more historically situated accounts to trace out the nature of the changes and what has influenced them. Here I can make common cause with the Caldwells' call for more culturally sensitive social research. My final comment remains the one that I began with: if we are to work at all with a model of a 'traditional' African morality, then its nature must be specified in a more tenable way. I hope that I have showed that in order to do this we must put marriage, respect and the religious values surrounding coitus back into the picture.

9

TRIBAL RITES AND TRIBAL RIGHTS

The first three chapters in this volume dealt with circumcision, that great pageant of ethnicity and manhood, which focuses on the heroism of its youth in standing this ordeal with the requisite bravery. It is an act of self-mortification, self-glorification and self-making. These chapters are all psychological in their discussion, as I enquire into the nature of manhood and how it is created in the ritual process. Circumcision is embodied identity at its most evident level, inscribed into the bodies of its Gisu men, just as it echoes through the landscape, through which it rings every two years, across the foothills and ridges of Mount Elgon, amid the deep green of the coffee plantations and banana groves.

In returning to the topic of circumcision, I do so to address further the question of ethnicity and of the power of 'tradition'. One aspect of Gisu nationhood, as indicated above, is the explicit way in which the tribal universe is envisioned in terms of masculinity. Nor are the Gisu alone in this for, in East Africa, they lie at one end of a broad belt of circumcising societies which stretches down from Mount Elgon through Kenya and into Tanzania. Not all groups within this geographic area circumcise but where they do it would be fair to say that the particular qualities of masculinity which it is seen to endow cannot easily be extricated from ethnic identity. Further, in Uganda, the Gisu hold themselves to be unique, with circumcision as their ethnic marker distinguishing them from all other peoples in Uganda, with the exception of the Sebei to their immediate north who, in addition, practise female clitoridectomy. The question posed starkly, then, is how does one particular 'custom' serve to mobilise collective sentiment in this one area and in this particular way?

Of tribe and tradition

As Ranger in his 1993 review of the topic explains, the idea of 'invented tradition' rapidly caught on in the academic world following the publication of Hobsbawm and Ranger's The Invention of Tradition (1983). And, not just in the specific sense used in the original, of traditions consciously crafted and adapted to suit new sets of circumstance, as, for example, in the new forms of pomp and ceremonial display in the colonialised worlds of the nineteenth and twentieth centuries. It caught on rather to explain all tradition. All, indeed, can be regarded as a product of invention, part of the artifice of culture, a product of the human imagination. But this current rendering fails to distinguish the different types of 'invention' or 'imaginings' – to use Anderson's (1983) term – we might be dealing with. The emphasis has been rather on the process of invention, with the detailed tracing of the historical – and largely political – forces which have shaped what is taken to be tradition.

One characteristic of identity and ethnicity in this region of East Africa – as others – is the constant play of differences, gradients of possibilities, realised differently. Each group has elaborated its own forms, out of a largely common stock, giving the impression of a Lévi-Straussian concern for différence. The peoples of this area to the north and the east of the Ugandan kingdoms of Buganda and Busoga were acephalous. Indeed, the Gisu on the western slopes of Mount Elgon, are part of a continuum of Bantu-speaking groups, speaking closely-related dialects, most of which are mutually intelligible. In Uganda, there are the Nyole, Gwere and Samia; to the East, across the border in Kenya, the large conglomeration of Luyia-speaking groups. Around this Bantu-speaking cluster – and in places interspersed with it – are Nilotic and Para-Nilotic speaking peoples; the Sebei to the north and separate groups of Teso to the north and east, the Padhola to the west, and so on. The 'tribe' as a bounded and exclusive unit should indeed be difficult to define. Indeed, within Bugisu, each clan, each sub-clan is known by its own 'customs' and dialect, the latter in some areas where the clans have streamed down from the mountains to the plains, varying each half a mile as one moves across the slopes of the Mountain.

One might think that this would provide classic ground for those current approaches to ethnicity which see it as a precipitate of its political history, more imposed from the outside than generated from within. Oral histories tell not of a fixed and settled past but of constant migrations, some temporary as in times of drought, others more permanent, as group vied with group for occupations of territory or small groups hived off from one area and intermarried into another. The picture of the pre-colonial past now is thus more of fuzzy boundaries and one might say fuzzy traditions, a collage of practice and form. This, despite their mountain base, is as true for the Gisu as for others, as the Gisu fought for occupancy of the plains with other peoples, and intermarried with them. Indeed, the practice of circumcision itself is traced to just such an instance of intermarriage, in this case of a Gisu man with a Nandi woman. Even the name Bagisu is said to be of foreign provenance, a Maasai praise name, derived from the Maasai word for cattle. This impression of flux and change would seem to provide the very conditions for the development of cultural identities formed as much in opposition to other groups as from an autonomous and innate sense of commonality.

Indeed, for some long while, the orthodoxy in African Studies with respect to tribal identifications is of colonial misunderstanding (if not deliberate guile in a policy of divide and rule) aided and abetted by anthropologists who gave a false cultural unity to the arbitrary units thus created. Early on, for example, Southall (1970) considered the Luyia a prime example of the influence of colonial rule in establishing tribal division, coming into being in the 1940s as a 'super-tribe', replacing the name used by the colonial administration for the area, Kavirondo, which had become opprobrious. Of interest here is that neither the Samia, whose population was cut in half by the national boundary between Uganda and Kenya nor the Gisu – linguistically just as close – have ever been regarded as Abaluyia and in the towns of East Africa both formed independent ethnic associations.

But, an externalist account of ethnicity only goes so far. Colonial boundaries as often as not, as the case above illustrates, mismatched the cultural units and, in so doing, created new ones; yet at the same time the local communities retained their own identities, unsubmerged. As Ranger says, such accounts 'really are very much first stage explanations. European classifications of race, or tribe or language in effect created a series of empty boxes, with bounded walls but without contents' (1993: 84). And there is more than a certain arbitrariness in such contents when looked at from a distance, drawn sometimes along one axis, sometimes another. The Gisu here would seem to lie at one end of a spectrum; at the end where one single practice equates with tribe. Elsewhere, the particular nature of ethnic identity is harder to define, perhaps little more than a common name, a mutually intelligible language, a myth of ancestry or of origin, a particular collection of customs or, more appropriately, of a set of ways of being human. None of this is well explained when seen simply as a fall-out from the facts of colonial rule. Indeed, such approaches sometimes seem but another twist on the theme of 'peoples without history', or for whom history is an effective by-product of an all-powerful and interventionist West. Thus, in shifting the emphasis to the political framing for the play of ethnicities, too often this identity has been seen solely as 'reactive'; whether this is in the form of collusion with or resistance to outside colonising processes.

Concerned with the way such interpretation underplays the extent of local initiative, a current generation of historians have given us more sophisticated accounts. The invention of ethnicities has come to be seen as a collaborative venture, a product of both external incentives and local interests and culture brokers. Thus, Chanock (1985), in his masterly study of colonial law in southern Africa, relates how the codification of customary law served to freeze the frame, reducing the uncertainty of an oral tradition, always in the making, dependent as often as not on might as much as right, to a fixed format of law and penalty. Colonialism created a new arena for discourse in which to talk of the customary legitimised claims to status, privilege and identity. The chiefs and new tribal authorities were quick to seize upon this aspect, as Chanock shows, and their courts and the laws they codified came to be seen as a repository of rights. Again from southern Africa, Leroy Vail (1997) singles out the experience of migrancy and the gendered nature of the tribal polity. He argues that, in the South African context, ethnic affiliation was fostered by a particular coalition of male interests which kept alive the links between rural and urban men, with its promise of control over both land and women.

These approaches have been concerned to show how the nature of ethnicity was changed – often dramatically – by the conditions of colonial rule. Far from being a pure residue of the past, ethnic tradition has come to be seen as a consciously crafted enterprise, which served the interests of power, whether of the colonisers, local rulers, or men as opposed to women. All these processes can be traced in Bugisu; there too a central authority gave notice of a cultural unity which could hardly have existed given the parochial nature of loyalties in the pre-colonial era. There too, the newly-elevated colonial chiefs set about enthusiastically formulating customary law in the courts and councils established in the 1920s. There too, there was labour migration – on a particularly massive scale in the inter-war years. Added to this, there were also important factors in the internal politics of the area. Interestingly, Bugisu was never an exclusive tribal enclave in the Colonial era, and its administrative identity changed at least five times, as it was incorporated into a district, first with one and then another of the surrounding areas. Only with Independence in 1963 did Bugisu become a unitary district. But this very lack of ethnic integrity may be adduced in turn to explain a growing awareness of 'tribe', as the district itself became a forum for competition and contest. One is mindful here of Lonsdale's (1992) stress on the importance of internal debate in the creation of ethnicity. Whether over land policy (in this desperately land-short area) or coffee marketing, there were many of these during the colonial period, and the issues have not declined in importance since then. Nevertheless, while all these factors might be important in detailing a growth in the formation of tribal conscious-ness, such a growth can only be assumed and, in any case, is insufficient in informing us about the source and power of this partic-ular imagining.

If recent commentaries have justly brought out the political and economic forces and the coalition of interests which have shaped the ethnicities of Africa during the colonial era, they have done scant justice to the meaningful. That one's ethnicity might be an important element in one's life chances, to a greater or lesser extent a negotiable asset for the individual trying to weave a way or make a viable living in today's multicultural world, with its intricate working of identities, is one thing. That it might provide the basis for political fault lines is another. Yet another is the subjective consciousness of it, its inward-looking aspects, which can be grasped but dimly through a concentration on its pragmatic uses. The emphasis on power has a tendency to vitiate all culture, emptying it of any value beyond protest, resistance or, even worse, some compensatory formation.

In this context, anthropologists need again to assert the vitality of local traditions of meaning, spinning out their own stories, in all the exigencies of the historical moment. Though Vansina (1990) discerns an abrupt dislocation between the old embedded traditions of Africa and the new world of modernising *mélange*, others are less pessimistic. Wendy James (1988) for the Uduk of the Sudan talks of a cultural archive, a sedimented layer of meaning upon which people draw in their task of creating and recreating themselves in line with the exigencies of history. And, this emphasis on the constant recreative powers of ordinary life, which transmutes custom in various ways, to ends both conscious and unconscious, must be one starting point. Lonsdale in his study of Mau Mau nationalism gives us another, stressing the creative achievement of ethnicity in itself, with Kikuyu nationalism seen as 'an intellectual response to social process' in which to 'debate civil virtue was to define ethnic identity' (1992: 268).

Feierman's (1990) stress on the role of the peasant intellectual also brings us back to the rural roots for the creation of meaning, and to the on-going task of interpretation and improvisation of tradition.

Interpretation, as always, must begin at home, with our own concepts. For, if the political scientists see the 'tribe' as a newly-formed artefact, a product of a fairly recent past, we have another set of problems when we turn to the concept of tradition, carrying the opposite implications – that of stasis. Never a technical term, nor one much used in anthropology, 'tradition' has come in as a surrogate, a circumlocution, a term more respectable than 'custom', apparently more precise than 'practice', but with its western connotations largely unexamined until recently. Even at its most neutral, the western picture of tradition is of a static form; a custom whose pattern is assumed to lie in the past, whose forms are followed even when their meanings are lost. It was in this context that the idea of 'invented traditions' came into prominence, cutting away the ground from an assumed authenticity, as one after another of such apparent traditions could be shown as relatively new and conscious creations.

If this were all, the concept would not be so pernicious but, additionally, for much social science, it continues to bear all the hallmarks of its Weberian heritage, and imply a particular 'psychic mind-set'. This involves a whole package of assumptions, hard to separate out from one another, as the concept of tradition is here linked to the idea of 'traditional societies'. Thus, to present a pastiche, the traditional worldview is held to be all-encompassing, authoritative, brooking no deviance or individual variation. Time-hallowed, people walk the same paths as their ancestors, looking to neither right nor left. Conformist and conservative, people not only resist change; they are unaware of any choice. As Popper put it, all critical or reflective thought is blocked, with people living in a 'charmed circle of unchanging taboos, of laws and customs which are felt to be as inevitable as the rising of the sun, or the cycle of the seasons' (1945: 57). This, in turn, is linked to a group versus an individual ethos; the individual in traditional societies is held to be so closely-bonded to his group and to its particular set of ascriptive social practices that he may hardly be said to exist apart from them.

As Mary Douglas (1982) has said, this myth bears no resemblance to anything that is known to anthropologists for its purpose, as she makes clear, has not been to illuminate the nature of these societies. It has been constructed to highlight by opposition the features taken to be distinctive of modern thought, and so we find bits and pieces of this picture finding their way into current discourses of modernity and postmodernity. In this context, Malinowski's (1926) diatribe against the picture of the native stuck in the grooves of immemorial tradition often seems as relevant today as it was seventy years ago. Unthinking conformity to a past pattern is foreign to the anthropological knowledge of the twentieth century. We would indeed have difficulties in explaining the dramatic transformations in the economic, legal and religious systems if we clung to the idea that people held some 'traditional' worldview that was inimical to such change.

One set of arguments here from anthropology has been the stress on the malleability of tradition in practice, the way in which an oral tradition allows for a ready manipulation of the past to serve diverse interests in the present. Again, to paraphrase Mary Douglas, cultural values are tactics as much as concepts, a view that renders all culture as the language of argument. My aim here is to make a rather different case by arguing that variation and choice might actually be built into the very concept of the 'traditional'. Thus, it is the ideology itself which, far from encouraging a passive acceptance of the 'nature of things', of 'fate', might actually encourage a pragmatic and even experimental attitude to it. Thus, it is not just that the practice, the easy alignment of past with present – what we might call the 'elision effect' – which readily allows for change, but that the ideologies of many 'traditional' peoples may themselves actively encourage it. Thus, we could say, the Gisu are traditional in the sense that their understanding of themselves, their identity as a people and as individuals, is given in the sense of continuity of the present with the past. But the nature of this tradition is highly specific and not at all like the 'traditionalism' of Western ideas. In the Gisu case, the idea of tradition does not imply a timeless template but actively incorporates both differentiation and change.

The most important practices of the Gisu, by which they define their sense of identity, indeed, which constitute their identity, are those of the *kimisambwa* (sing: *kumusambwa*). These are the vectors of ancestral continuity and it is these which, at first glance, one is most tempted to translate as traditions – ancestral traditions. A more faithful translation, however, would be ancestral powers or forces, for these operate not by an insistence on a passive conformity to rules laid down but by their active interventions in human life. They 'catch' those who fall within their orbit. Initially, their characteristic sign is that of affliction, each being associated with a known range of symptoms, which can then be brought under control through rituals which both cure and, importantly, empower the individual, aligning him or her with the particular ancestral force. Some clearly have a 'totemic' aspect, being associated with animals, birds, or other features of the natural environment. Others are more occupational in appearance for all the more important Gisu specialisations are included within this category: divination, rainmaking, smithing, and of course, most significantly, the power of the circumcisers and of circumcision itself, the *kumusambwa kw'imbalu.*

The first point to be noted here is their tremendous variation for their distribution varies throughout Bugisu in an essentially non-systematic way. The Gisu, in fact, recognise only the one *kumusambwa* which holds for all Gisu, that of male circumcision. For the rest, the particular way circumcision is performed is subject to considerable regional variation and variation over time, as people modify, elaborate and embroider upon their own particular ceremonials. As the focus for cultural interests, gripping the imagination, as does no other, it is also the arena for the greatest cultural innovation. New elements follow hard and fast upon one another.

The point to be made is that this constant innovation poses no threat to the Gisu concept of tradition. There is no sense in which this is an example of 'invented traditions'. That only has a meaning in terms of a concept which assumes that a practice laid down in a particular form in the past acts as an authoritative template for the present and future. For the Gisu there is nothing ever entirely fixed about the form for the continuity with the past is given not only in *what* things are handed on but rather more in *how* they are. To put it in other words, it is about the mechanism as much as the content. The mechanism is that of ancestral transmission. The *kimisambwa* perpetuate themselves by catching people within their orbit; they thus follow kinship. The unchanging nature of ancestral tradition derives from this; it is seen to continue down the generations with the same strength. But, which ancestral powers people are subject to is variable and to some extent contingent, for the constellation of kinship varies for all, over time and over space, and so do the *kimisambwa.* Ancestral powers – and the particular sets of ritual restrictions and imperatives (*kimisiro*) with which they are associated – wax and wane as they are brought into different relationships with each other over time; each marriage creating a different set of possibilities for the future.

Custom, understood in this way, is open and fluid and not static and fixed. This is true throughout and, because of this lability, which *kimisambwa* are actually in force for particular people is often difficult to specify. Indeed, in many instances, they are essentially unknowable. They can be known only through experience, and this, if only in a superficial sense, renders Gisu attitudes to their custom experimental in nature. To give an example, when I was first in the field, I was bewildered by the variety in the marriage rules people gave me. Even people of the same small lineage would give me different degrees of consanguinity as marking the effective boundaries for marriage or incest. My first clue as to how to interpret this came when an old man said, well, he knew what the rules had been when he was young but he did not know what people could do today. Now, this was not an instance of social change, of the effects of modernisation disrupting some accepted traditional order. Matter of fact, it was spoken with no sense of disapproval, and he went on to elaborate upon how his father's sister had married a distant cousin within formerly prohibited degrees and she had not only lived but flourished and now had eight children. The rule thus had presumably changed. I then went back to people who had told me that they could not marry so closely and, sure enough, they all had their own precedents: their aunts had tried it out but far from succeeding had met with disaster and infertility. The lessons were clear in all cases but in none of them was it a lesson which could be generalised to others.

The distinctive nature of everyone's kinship make its rules particularistic. But this is not all. Not only is there the recognised fact of variation but, because of the way in which ancestry and the *kimisambwa* operate, you can never be quite sure which rules are in fact in operation – at least for you. The fact that other people in your kindred have been caught by the power of divination, of the leopard, or of rainmaking, for example, makes it no more than a possibility that you will. What holds then, in a sense, can be tested out only in action. Indeed, we can perhaps go further. Among the Gisu, the idea of an ancestrally-derived order and rules allows – and even invites – a testing out of what is and what is not in force. The operative principle is uncertainty. One can never know for sure which rules are in operation and circumstances frequently lead one individual or another to take a chance, break a taboo, disregard custom, in the hope or even the expectation that the boundaries might have shifted. And this pragmatic questioning attitude is carried over to much of what goes on in their lives, as for example, is seen with respect to divination (see Chapter Six).

The Gisu then show little of the reverential attitude to 'tradition' that the 'model', admittedly something of a straw man, might lead us to expect. Nor, of course, is this unique in the ethnographic record which abounds in examples of people changing their marriage rules or system of property transmission, often over night, and with few qualms, just as they have adopted Christianity in many and various forms, experimenting with ideas as, or even more, freely than with the technological innovations that came with colonialist expansion. Yet, ancestrally-transmitted, the very features which allow for its continuing evolution, also explain its tenacity. Circumcision cannot die. Nor, can it be allowed to lest, it is said, the Gisu themselves die out. This might be taken as an appropriate metaphoric rendering of the power of this collective identity, but it is given more concrete form in the belief that the shade of an uncircumcised man will return to destroy his entire kindred. Such dead are attributed with uncontrollable malevolence and, whether one looks upon this as legitimisation or fear, it is this which lies behind the circumcision 'task forces' that take it upon themselves to round up boys who have dallied too long and, where necessary, forcibly circumcise them. This occurs both within the District and in the towns of East Africa and during the biennial circumcision periods the newspapers usually carry at least one 'horror' story, often involving a claim of mistaken identity with a non-Gisu youth being cut. It is in this context that I turn to the recent case of Kabala.

Tribal rites and human rights

If this chapter, up to now, has been about the power of tradition, this takes another form when we consider the rights of the individual in relation to the group. The question of human rights has raised its head most strongly with respect to female circumcision or clitoridectomy, in its many and various forms. Throughout this century, Westerners, whether missionaries or feminists, have had no problem with defining this practice as destructive, cruel, even as an 'atrocity'. Combined with a vision that such rites service a patriarchal culture, their apparently voluntary aspect on the part of women can then be seen as a forced rather than as a free choice. I don't wish to add more words to this debate, as my point is simply to highlight that male circumcision, with its Biblical precedents, has never been condemned in the same way. Medical textbooks may indeed debate its merits but it is popularly regarded as non-problematic, on the easy assumption that such a widespread social practice, even where it has no particular religious meaning has other, particularly hygienic, benefits. So, one operation is rendered harmful, the other harmless, even positively beneficial. Such a view, of course, largely disregards the varying severity of the operation itself and the mode of operation. And, it disregards the human rights implications which are possibly no different from those raised by female clitoridectomy.

'Are you free to denounce your tribe?' asked the feature in the Ugandan publication *The New Vision* in January 1995. Duallo wa Chibita goes on to ask, 'Does a person who desires to opt out of his culture have any protection under the law? What happens when the rights of an entire tribe clash with those of an individual member of that tribe? Whose rights will prevail?' This article – and a series of others – was prompted by the dramatic actions of Kabala who, to evade the threat of the circumcision task forces, went to the lengths of registering a new tribe, in which he was the founding – and possibly still – the sole member. Finding no redress under Ugandan Law, Kabala, a Makerere University student, took the opportunity while attending a conference in Toronto, Canada, to contact Marcus Garvey's Universal Negro Improvement Association. They assisted him in incorporating his new multi-national tribe, the Khaluba – with its own language, a mixture of Luo, Bantu and Russian – under both Canadian Provincial and Federal Law. There are three proposed criteria for membership. Firstly, those of black descent who wish to be legally identified as Africans. Second, any person who is a prisoner of conscience and wishes to renounce repugnant cultural practices of their origin and thirdly, those who cannot trace their ancestral lineage due to intermarriage or migration and wish to 'establish a family of association and identification'. This new tribe was brought into being on 30th December 1994.

This might be thought of as a prime instance of how globalising factors are operating to open up the sphere of choice for 'local subjects'. But though there is novel action here, we can also trace strong lines of continuity. Firstly, the appeal to international organisations is hardly unprecedented in Africa. Indeed, Marcus Garvey's movement, established in 1914, has long provided recourse for Africans in search of their rights and in search of religious validation. It proved particularly powerful in southern Africa in the first half of this century, providing a source of support and inspiration for several generations of religious leaders, who brought back to Africa the ideals of self-respect for their African heritage that Garvey promulgated (Sundkler, 1948). The fact that Kabala came from a Seventh Day Adventist family may also be relevant since throughout East Africa it is they who are at the forefront of resistance to tribal practices seen as an anathema to their faith.[1]

However, Kabala is not the first Gisu to wish to evade the ordeal. Indeed, he came from a family of escapees. His father, Mafaabi, left Bugisu in his youth to work as a teacher in Buganda where he married a Ganda wife and brought up his children without teaching them

Lugisu. Mafaabi evaded the operation until 1982 when, to escape Museveni's bush war, he returned to the Gisu town of Mbale. There – at sixty years of age – he was caught and publicly circumcised. In addition to this, as Kabala put it, his uncle had also been subjected to degrading treatment, by being circumcised after his death at the burial site, a normal Gisu practice in such cases. And, Kabala himself, during his years as a student, had been repeatedly threatened by the circumcision 'task forces'. He had motive enough to detest a 'tribe' to which he had never claimed any allegiance.

Clearly, in such circumstances we are not just faced with people at a cross-roads, unsure which direction to take, but we are involved with a battle of faiths, even of fundamentalisms. The choices in such cases could hardly be further from the transposable, pick-and-mix identities talked of for the 'late modern' citizen (Hall, 1996). Rather, they are dealing with difficult moral dilemmas in carving out a space to live. Kabala acted in a novel way, but he was acting in terms of East African cultural idioms. He didn't just reject his tribe; he did it in the only effective way given the circumstances – by affiliating himself to another.

As Lonsdale says the tribe provides 'a layer of meaning that academics find difficult to discuss' (1992:110). And, he points out that the opposite is true in East Africa where it remains the cardinal principle of identity and, if its crunch time comes earlier with the Gisu than with other tribes, everyone is involved in the moral debates that it brings in train. Is one free to reject it? The issue is one that fires public opinion in the way no other does, as the burial case of S.M. Otieno of 1986/87 in Kenya so vividly showed. It is worth saying a few words to indicate the parallels here. In this burial case – not the first or last in Kenya, but possibly the most sensational to date – the issue was again prompted by a mixed marriage, with Otieno, a prominent Luo lawyer having married Wambui, from an elite Kikuyu family. Put simply, the fight over the corpse and where it should be buried was fought out between the rights of the tribal lineage to bury their own person and the rights claimed by the wife as 'next of kin'. The battle contested through the courts, all the way to appeal, was followed through every twist and turn by an avid reading public. Ultimately the 'tribe' was declared the winner, and the body was transported back to Luoland for burial 155 days after his death, a decision which many saw as a conservative reiteration of patriarchal culture.

Yet, as the many commentators on this case have pointed out, what exactly it was all about runs so thickly through the various strands of the national culture, that it defies a simple summary. It seemed at the time to be about everything that really mattered to the Kenyan people; the clash of rights created by kinship versus marriage, of rural versus urban life, of old men versus new men, of tribal beliefs versus Christianity, of oral versus literate culture, of the division between non-circumcising and circumcising peoples, of Luo versus Kikuyu; clashes which cannot, given the complexities of the case, simply be summarised as those of tradition versus modernity. But running throughout all of them, and to a large extent echoing all these lines of cleavage, was the opposition of men to women. We certainly all became aware, if we hadn't before, of just how masculine tribal law had been and still was.

The question of who a person belongs to, and thus what are the appropriate customary forms in the new situations which confront them, is a question that concerns everyone. In the Luo case, it seemed that the decisive moment of affiliation is death. But these issues are being played out on the national stage. Indeed, Cohen and Odhiambo even see the case as a 'significant moment in the construction of a Kenya nation' (1992: 92). Certainly, it is the national law which is being made and remade by such cases. The Kabala case, though it inspired headlines in the national papers, fired a more direct challenge at only one of its many cultures. Evidently, it was the talk only of Mbale town, the Gisu capital – something which reiterates the importance of the internal rather than the external debate in the play of construction and reconstruction of ethnic identities.

In Uganda, there was no national court case. The clause built into the colonial law with respect to its customary forms still holds and allows them to be applied as long as they are not repugnant with equity, natural justice and good conscience.[2] Yet, Kabala could find no lawyer to act for him, partly because of the difficulties of arguing that the practice, which is an injunction in Islam and Judaism and often advocated for medical reasons, is 'repugnant' in itself. Nor can an injunction easily be taken out against unspecified members of the circumcision task forces who operate in the towns. A prosecution for assault thereafter would be, one can easily see, too late. Legally fighting over a deceased corpse is one thing, fighting over an intact foreskin, perhaps, is another. No doubt there will come a time when such cases are referred to International Courts of Human Justice and one wonders then how the lawyers will resolve the issue of the rights of the individual versus the collective, and how they will deal with the particular nature of Gisu tradition. But, for the moment, the power of the lawyers has not reached into the Bugisu mountains and the arbiters of the issue remained local and national.

The more interesting question might be, how many will follow

Kabala into his new tribe? On the face of it, it seems unlikely that his case will spell a wholesale flight from circumcision, a rejection of identity. Gisu men have been fleeing circumcision for some time – perhaps always. Running away is the most obvious course of action but, to resume a Gisu identity, to take up residence again in the district, such men must return to be cut. During circumcision time, it was a not uncommon sight to see such returnees. One particular instance from 1966 still stands out in my memory. I was talking to an elder in one of the ancestral groves in a mountainous area of Central Bugisu a week or so before the main rituals were due to begin. While there, we saw a middle-aged man, in full city rig, furled umbrella and briefcase, being marched purposefully along the path, flanked on each side by two local men in the more usual garb of shorts and shirts. It was an incongruous sight and I turned to ask the reason. The elder indicated that I should wait: all would become clear. As indeed it did, for on arrival at the nearest homestead, the circumcision shout went up immediately. This man had, it was then explained, left Bugisu in his youth and had been working in Nairobi as a civil servant. He had come back prepared, knowing what awaited him.

The other option, also available for the last fifty years, has been circumcision in a hospital. While this evasion does not bestow any honour, 'you cannot be cut twice', as the Gisu say, and it is usually regarded as acceptable for educated boys. What is interesting in the Kabala case is the open defiance, the head-on collision course, fired by the particular circumstances of his family, by his non-Gisu upbringing, by his religious convictions. And, perhaps, as these circumstances become more common, others will follow Kabala. It is worth noting here that the other evasive options were in the past mainly exercised by the educated elite, though probably never in great numbers and never totally restricted to them.

But the fact that there have always been escapees has another side to it as well which, far from threatening Gisu self-conceptions, reinforces them. Insofar as it operates to highlight fearfulness of the ordeal, it correspondingly reinforces the heroism of those who 'voluntarily' choose it – and then succeed, of course. Even the long build-up to the operation, which I once saw – and still do – as a form of battleproofing (see Chapter Three), preparing the initiates for their test, can, from another angle, be seen to make failure more likely, since it constantly harps on it, holding it out as a possibility. Clearly, pre-operative rituals are not essential for the success of such operations and, in fact, are comparatively rare in the Kenyan context. Yet, the boys (and the girls too) are expected to be just as stoic, indeed, to the point where the possibility of failure is almost totally denied. In Bugisu, however, they can and do fail; in extreme cases polluting their homestead and the circumcision knife. I thus now begin to appreciate how the ritual might prepare not just for success but also for failure.

Wangusa's novel, *Upon this Mountain*(1989), gives a further insight into the cultural patterning at issue here. On the very day of circumcision, a few men parade as women, provoking much ribald humour, all good fun. For many years, I wondered about the meaning of this. How, on a day dedicated to the making of men, could men ape femininity? Was this a ritual of rebellion? Did it express rejection or resentment of the male role (an almost immediate explanation where women cross-dress during rituals)? Well, this would have to be at some deep – very deep – level and, even then, it didn't seem likely. Wangusa's story, however, contains an account of a boy who fails the ordeal, and the story continues with the narrator later meeting him, now permanently dressed as a woman. A very much more obvious interpretation of the transvestite behaviour on circumcision day, therefore, is that it operates – whether consciously or unconsciously – as a taunt and warning to the boy. And, it gives notice also of the fact that the Gisu too have their 'third gender', an African variant of the *berdache*.[3] There are men who are permanently accepted as transsexuals, donning women's clothes and classifying as 'women'. I became aware of them at funerals where they acted as funeral drummers, a role said to be the preserve of women. No one ever linked this pattern to a circumcision failure; the explanation invariably proffered was pragmatic. Having a female identity was one way of avoiding paying one's taxes!

We thus have in Bugisu a good – perhaps classic – form of hegemonic masculinity, in the sense of a dominant model, defined in terms that apparently brook no contradiction all the way to the grave. Yet, the Gisu also have their variant or subordinate forms, and were tolerant of both transsexuality and homosexuality. True it was a stigmatised activity, especially shameful for men who took the 'female role', but was treated with amused contempt, rather than shock, horror and sanction. One could say perhaps that it was not an issue – at least one never felt it as such then. Rather, the issues of moral debate concerned those men who had proved their manhood by standing the ordeal but then failed to live up to its terms, as detailed in Chapter Five.

This alerts us once again to the complexity of gender relations as the apparently obvious inferences may lead us astray. The valorisation of masculinity in this case allows not for a sharply dichotomised gender division, but introduces a third term, an identity stigmatised to be sure but liveable. Further, circumcision itself does not act to totally oppose the genders (see further Chapter Four) for women share in its ritual and indeed in its valour. Indeed, in many ways, it can be regarded as a rite of passage for girls as well, as they stand by their brothers during the climateric of the last three days and are cleansed together with them by the circumciser after the operation.

Nevertheless, in conclusion, I should say more about the particular construction of Gisu gender divisions and sexuality. This topic is now at the forefront of academic writing, with the discourses of sexuality seen as deeply imbricated with power relationships. One particular image that brings this question to mind is that many years after my fieldwork among the Gisu, I heard in Kenya the striking metaphor of the 'sharpened spear'. This was used specifically of the circumcised penis, carrying with it the idea that the penis was forged and fashioned not only against men in battle but against women in sexual combat. The powerfulness of the idea is clear enough, catching in one image the nature of masculinity in male conquest and female defeat, supremacy and subordination and the *agonis* of gender relationships. Women here can never be 'on top' – and this is reinforced by a cultural behaviour set which ensures that women are always literally lower than men, whether ducking in their presence or sitting on the ground while the men claim the chairs. Further, this aspect is very widespread in East Africa so that even the poet, Okot p'Bitek (1973) in writing of the Acholi – who, it should be stressed, do not circumcise – shows that a similar imagery in courtship prevails there, where the young men 'shoot' the girls they desire.

The extent to which, worldwide, the sexual act is rendered culturally as an act of aggression undoubtedly varies. In Kenya, it reaches its most extreme expression possibly among the Gusii, for whom LeVine (1959) wrote that all sexual intercourse was played as rape, with women even in marriage expected to resist. He was moved to write this article because of the persistently high rates of reported rape in that area, stretching back through the colonial period. More recently, in July 1991, the Kenyan public was stunned by the boys' rape of the girls at a boarding school in another district of Kenya, that of Meru, which resulted in the death of nineteen girls. The horror of this event prompted calls – especially by women's organisations – for public debate on gender violence and the general harassment and inequality suffered by Kenyan women. It was a call which was only partially heard for, terrible as this tragedy was, the Government authorities seem to have acted to suppress it, with only two of the many boys involved ever charged, and then only with rape.[4] Rioting in schools, in itself, has become commonplace, and it seems as if boys' dissatisfactions and frustrations with their school authorities are readily transposed onto girls who become the 'enemy'. If the tragedy in Meru was a singular event, the attitudes which led to it are more widespread. In such a context the metaphor of the 'sharpened spear' is anything but innocent.

That manhood had two linked attributes among the Gisu – warrior-hood and sexuality – I had realised; that they might be joined together in such a way, I had not. My immediate response was to think that I might have overlooked this aspect and I rushed back to my fieldnotes to see if they provided any evidence for this imaging of sexual desire. I couldn't find it. Indeed, the lack of overt sexual symbolism in the circumcision ritual is a feature that I take up in Chapter Four as it is one that almost forces a psychoanalytic perspective. Now that I have worked in Kenya, I am even more sharply aware of the differences, for the attitudes that LeVine talks of for the Gusii of forty years ago could pass as a description for their neighbours, the Kuria of today. I say this in order to say that, on balance, I think that I got it 'right': in Bugisu it is the military role of circumcision which is stressed and the element of sexual dominance played down. Sex here was not 'played' – to use an East African idiom – in a way that assumes that men alone emerge as victors.[5]

This is in accord with the *real politik* of gender relationships here – where men's control over their wives is more formal than real. Gisu women were not powerless. They were not, as they were among the Gusii (and to a large extent among the Kuria also), 'stranger' wives, dependent upon the goodwill of husband and mother-in-law. Usually, Gisu wives came from neighbouring families, with a good contingent of brothers and fathers to keep a watchful eye on their affairs. And, they expected to be the immediate mistresses of their own house, not a subservient member of a large homestead. Further, Gisu women were relatively free to divorce and remarry and thus, despite a jural situation which appeared to deny them rights, in practice they had a strong bargaining hand in relationship to their husbands. One was far more aware of men's fears about the loyalty of their wives than of women mercilessly exploited by brutal husbands.

Yet, both of these stands mingle in the gender politics of East Africa, with its images of loose women and hard men. And so, it is worth saying something of that other important category of escapees – the women. In the 1960s, Gisu welfare associations in Nairobi from time to time, railed back their 'wayward women' who could be seen parading around Mbale for a day or two. Their numbers, their mini-skirted attire and their insouciance clearly distinguished them from the normal run of women, who were there on a thousand errands and mindful of the need to catch the bus home. But, these 'new' women soon melted away, back most probably to the towns from which they had been so summarily 'deported'. Other women returned in one's and two's, summoned back sometimes because of a family crisis, and sometimes by being tricked into thinking that there was one. Many of these women were those who had left their husbands but never returned to the parental home, a common ruse in those days since, until the woman returned to her father, he was under no obligation to return the bridewealth. As this reminds us, we have to be careful of automatically interpreting female migration to towns as an act of female liberation, a fleeing from the demands of patriarchal culture. As White's (1990) study of prostitution in Nairobi so clearly shows, many of the women who flocked to Nairobi at various times during the colonial period, were not so much in search of liberty but were essentially compensating for the poverty of their menfolk in the rural areas, and it was to these men that they returned, together with their earnings. Indeed, given the freedom of Gisu women within Bugisu, one wonders if the deportation committees in Nairobi were not fired more by the kind of ethnic shame generated in that town by its many 'loose' women rather than to factors nearer home. But, that speculation can only be an aside.

The common Kenyan (indeed African) expression that women have no tribe refers at its most evident to the fact that 'tribe' is no barrier to marriage as women take on their husband's tribal affiliations. Yet it also indicates the key perception that tribal orders are masculine orders and that in thinking about tribal divisions in East Africa men think of them in terms of other men and other manhoods. In this attitude, women are deemed irrelevant. However, clearly, it does not mean that the 'tribe' does not claim them – or rather that particular men do not – for if men have 'tribe', a large part of the rights this bestows are over women. And the idea of women without tribes takes on another ring in the modern age as women seek and earn new freedoms outside the tribal enclaves, posing an evident threat to male power and control. The Otieno case at one level was about tribal (moral) man versus modern (immoral) woman. And, in this context, one is tempted to ask whether rituals such as circumcision for men have not gained in symbolic valency over the course of this century for this very reason. As we have learnt to see, tribal rites translate into tribal rights.

As La Fontaine (1977) so memorably argued, Gisu *imbalu* can be seen to be about the 'power of rights' and, from this viewpoint, it is relevant to ask how far circumcision now has to do double duty in defining manhood, as men have lost their former military role and their control over women comes increasingly also under threat? Just as women's liberties have evident consequential effects on men's, so do the changes in the political economy, which have undercut male autonomy in the rural areas, forcing more and more of them into the marginal worlds of the city to scrape a living in increasingly hard economic times. If men retreat into 'tribe' as the source of rights, then their right to it, maybe, can only be asserted through such a stress on initiation and thereafter in an exercise of their 'manhood' for which control over women remains for many the tangible sign.

But, as everywhere, the institutional features – the features which differ from locality to locality – are as important as the overall cultural themes or economic factors which shape the regional scene. Here, I return to the Gisu and reiterate the fact that the uncompromising nature of Gisu manhood comes to the fore in direct competition among men for control over resources. Circumcision gives men rights to citizenship and to the economic resources that go with it – but, to an extent, they must still be won. These resources, both land and women, in the Gisu context pit men against men and not men against women. It is no sign of masculinity in the Bugisu hills for men to rape and kill women. Not only were both rare but a man's rights over the person of his wife did not include the right to beat her, and women took cases out against their husband when this occurred. In this, as I have said, they contrast with many others of the East African cultures. And, as an anthropologist, let me stress the long historical precedence for this, and the importance of understanding locality, as a source not only for the power of rights but for its limitations and permutations over time.

Moving from a concern with the power of tradition, the last half of this chapter has taken up a series of *causes célèbres* which illustrate current issues of ethical debate in the eastern African context. In one way or another, they all deal with the rights claimed in the name of groups over the individual, rights which extend over the bodies of their citizens, whether male, female, alive or dead. The cases created dramatic foci for the contestation of rights, insights into the politics of identity and into the power of the categorical divisions which construct the realm of the social. Cutting across diverse areas of social concern, the issues of human rights and women's rights were brought to the fore against those of the collective male. It would be conventional to say that such debates are formative in the construction of new identities, providing new as well as old axes for identification, new as well as old arguments and alignments of interest. And, no doubt this is true. But, the aspect that they all attest to, though in varying ways, is the continuing strength of local affiliation. Despite all the forces of modernity, the 'tribe' shows no signs of withering away. And, perhaps, in time, this stubborn fact will cease to be an academic embarrassment. In the shifting perspective of today, where once the 'tribe' was seen solely as a negative force, a counter to the integrative powers of the nation, it is as likely to be reinterpreted in a more positive light, as a local counter to the all-encompassing powers of the global.

In this context, one should stress again that Gisu circumcision is not just about an ever-receding past but about the contemporary moment. Discourses of masculinity and belonging are still dominant. Though the modern theorists of identity tell us (uncontroversially) that all identities are constructed in difference, the corresponding denial of identity as formed in shared experience does not necessarily follow. The Gisu imagining of their identity as male citizens is deeply 'essentialist' and, while it might be thought that the strength and formation of this male character had much to do with a militaristic past, its continuing salience can just as easily be related to the very loss of a warrior role. No simple anachronism, it keeps it alive as a possibility, and provides the discursive justification for male claims to status. And, as I have been concerned to show throughout these chapters, this, in turn, creates its own characteristic moral dilemmas.

NOTES

2 THE MAKING OF MEN: THE RELEVANCE OF VERNACULAR PSYCHOLOGY TO THE INTERPRETATION OF A GISU RITUAL

I am grateful to Paul Heelas, Audrey Richards and Jean Smith for their encouragement and critical comments on an earlier version of this chapter

. 1 The Gisu are a Bantu-speaking people who inhabit the western slopes of Mount Elgon. The rich soils of this extinct volcano support a dense population, with densities rising to 1,500 to the square mile in the more mountainous regions. The staple crops are plantain and millet while arabica coffee and cotton provided the main cash income during the 1960s.

2 See La Fontaine 1957, 1967 and 1969.

3 Particularly Geertz, 1957, 1966 and 1973.

4 e.g. Richards, 1956a, 1967 and 1970. In 1956, Richards widened the analysis of puberty rituals to include psychological utility, what she called the 'pragmatic effects' of ritual. The later articles contain a fuller assessment of the implications of the neglect of the individual and of the wider Malinowskian concern with values that has characterised British social anthropology.

5 La Fontaine, in an initial concern with participants' terms, in fact goes some way towards the position advocated in this chapter. I fully appreciate her view that 'initiation rituals create occasions in which traditional wisdom is communicated, tested and vindicated', but am less happy with the corollary that this is the 'source of the power of rights' (1977: 434). Deriving from a structuralist concern with social classification she argues that the rituals should be seen as a way of maintaining discrete social divisions. In the Gisu case she argues that this is achieved through the establishment of an opposition between youths and elders: power predicated on physical strength versus authority predicated on knowledge. While a full discussion of her complex argument is outside the province of this chapter it is necessary to register disagreement with the thrust of an interpretation which tends to see Gisu circumcision as primarily acting to validate authority, specifically the authority of elders.

6 The following account is based on fieldwork carried out in the Central and Southern regions of Bugisu between September 1965 and May 1969. During this time I was fortunate enough to be able to witness and follow through two entire circumcision periods (1966 and 1968). In addition, in 1968, with Richard Hawkins and his team from the UCLA Ethnographic Film Unit, I helped to make film of the ceremonies which takes up the story of two boys from the time they decide upon the ordeal. The focus taken by the film profoundly influenced the way I saw the ceremonies and it vividly illustrates some of the themes of this chapter (see Hawkins and Heald, 1988).

7 Since my first aim in this chapter is to give an understanding of Gisu attitudes to circumcision I translate the Gisu term *umusinde* as 'candidate' or 'boy' in preference to the more technical-sounding 'novice' or 'initiand'. *Umusinde* has the normal meaning of 'boy'. 'Candidate' is, however, the translation usually chosen by English-speaking Gisu who thus put the emphasis on the idea of a person undergoing a test.

8 In one particular area of Bugisu, in the mountains of southern Bugisu which border Kenya, the ceremonies of some clans take a rather different form and somewhat younger boys are circumcised. La Fontaine has stressed the wide variation in dialect and ritual practices within Gisu society which serve as differentiating features. Thus, 'the same symbols, invoked with reference to their details, may divide where their general characteristics may serve as the rallying point for tribal unity' (1969: 189). With reference to the ceremonies, the most significant divide which has a bearing on the description offered here is that between the mountainous regions of Central and Southern Bugisu where collective lineage-based rituals are held and the rest of Bugisu where the ceremonials tend to be less elaborate in form. Where rites are distinctive to the former areas this is indicated in the text.

9 In the situation of sacrifice the heart and the organs associated with the breath and the voice – the lungs and two top ribs – are hung on the forked stick of the shrine erected for the ancestors. This is said to show that 'we have given the whole of the animal' – its life, strength and dispositions.

10 This quotation comes from the film *Imbalu* (see Hawkins and Heald, 1988) where the situation is clearly depicted.

11 These stages differ from those described by La Fontaine (1959), and followed by Turner (1969), in that three stages rather than four are discriminated in this account and greater significance is given to beer brewing and the way in which the novice himself inaugurates each stage.

12 La Fontaine's interpretation of such trances as involving the loss of physical control, irresponsibility and general unawareness of events runs counter to the interpretation given here. Where such trance behaviour occurs – and it is by no means universal – I see it as indicating total identification with the ordeal and thus not indicative of any loss of control, either mental or physical. Compare here La Fontaine (1977: 426–27) on the novices 'blundering about' with the dangers consequent upon such loss of physical control (especially pp. 16–17); and on the impact of the addresses of the elder on the initiates (ibid.: 429; cf. 19).

13 Space precludes further consideration of the link between wildness and the ancestors but it can be noted that other actions tend also to identify the

boy with the non-social, placing him apart from normal domestic routine. For example, in one rite the boy does not cut down branches of plantains but knocks them down with his fists and in carrying water for his beer he must balance the pot on his head without the aid of a head-rest.

14 There is debate over writing Lugisu as the dialects vary considerably throughout Bugisu. In this book, I transcribe Gisu words according to the pronunciation of the central/southern dialect. Thus, I write *lirima* rather than *litima*, as la Fontaine writes it following the northern pronunciation. In addition, I also use some phonetic symbols; 'x' refers to the velar fricative, usually written 'kh' in Uganda, and 'c' to the palative fricative which is pronounced as the 's' in sugar.

15 One of the difficulties in dealing with this area is the lack of a one-to-one correlation between 'emotion' and physiological stimulus. As Schachter has shown there is a necessary cognitive dimension to emotional experience so that a given physiological input is not in itself sufficient to create the appropriate emotional affect (Schacter and Singer, 1962). The point of interest in the Gisu concept of *lirima* is perhaps that it draws attention not to a specific emotion but rather to the intensity of response, making a physiological correlation perhaps more appropriate. See further, Chapter Three of this volume.

16 Applying the symbolic interactionist learning theory of G.H. Mead, Kapferer argues that in certain healing rites 'the ritual organisation of symbolic action and content in performance reveals a process whereby the Self is constructed and reconstructed' (1979: 130). He suggests that a similar perspective might illuminate the transformational dynamics of *rites of passage*. Without using the specific terminology associated with Mead and his followers this paragraph indicates what such an interpretation might imply for the Gisu rites.

17 Fears of cursing and retributive action by the ancestral ghosts are associated not so much with how the boy stands the operation but rather with his fate afterwards and are frequently resorted to in explaining failures in early adult life (see further, Chapter Five and Heald, 1998).

18 V.W. Turner's 1969 article on Gisu circumcision is explicitly concerned with the analysis of these three substances, claiming that a key to their central meaning 'is to be found by considering them in their operational social setting and in their processual character as both indices and agencies of change in the structure of social relations' (202–03). The primacy here given to the structural dimension has led to some unlikely symbolic interpretations as La Fontaine has made clear (La Fontaine, 1972: notes 12 and 26)

19 See further, Horton (1960), Goody (1961) and Peel (1969).

20 'Reflexive' in the sense outlined by I. A. Richards (1936) and Polanyi and Prosch (1975) in their work on the power of metaphor.

21 La Fontaine (1977: 429) and I both see these three substances as analogues in the context of circumcision. It is, however, important to mention that chyme, which is used in many ritual contexts carries also connotations of purification and blessing. To this extent its meaning could be said to be wider than that of the other two substances. The mud, *litosi*, used for circumcision is used in no other ritual context and, interestingly, where yeast is used in other situations it seems to carry a similar incitement to

violent emotion. One other prominent example of the ritual use of yeast is at funerals where the close female relatives daub their faces with yeast and, waving pangas, loudly lament the death as they lead the other mourners in the funeral dances.

22 It is possible that such a tension exists in all religious beliefs. As has been seen, the terms of the contrast conform in essentials to those which have been the subject of debate between the Durkheimian 'symbolists' represented by Beattie and the Tylorian 'literalists' championed by Horton. It may, however, be more pronounced in those African cosmologies which, like that of the Gisu, see the individual as being at the centre of a field of interacting forces and thus vulnerable to 'outside' influence, yet at the same time recognise the discreteness of the person and place strong emphasis on individual responsibility. The circumcision rituals give very definite expression to this tension and different emphases are apparent at different phases of the rite. Thus, the stress on individual responsibility and control of the pre-operative phase contrasts with the loss of such autonomy. The post-operative situation where recovery is attributed to external influences and, as has been dealt with in detail here, both aspects are present during the climacteric of the three-day operation period.

23 As La Fontaine (1977) has noted, some of the ritual restrictions gain their significance from this association of procreation and fermentation. During the three-day fermentation period the people making the beer should refrain from sexual intercourse lest they 'spoil' the beer, making it in this case 'too strong'. La Fontaine in commenting upon this says, 'In this context brewing and sexual intercourse are antitheses which must be separated' (1977: 430). I would, however, argue that, based on an underlying cosmology of interacting forces, it is sympathy and not antipathy which is at issue; the fear being that the powers released during intercourse will positively augment those present in the beer, so intensifying fermentation. A similar sympathetic principle has been noted in the action of the smearing substances on the boy. After circumcision, when the boy is in a contrasting ritual phase, devoid of *lirima*, both sexual intercourse and pregnancy alike are believed to pose a direct danger to him. Then he must be protected from any such excitation in his immediate environment lest his curing be retarded. Thus it is of critical importance that none of the wives of the elder in whose home he is curing is pregnant and that all in the homestead refrain from sexual intercourse during the period of the boy's healing, normally until the final aggregation ceremonies some four or five months later.

24 Especially Turner, 1967.

3 THE RITUAL USE OF VIOLENCE:
CIRCUMCISION AMONG THE GISU OF UGANDA

1 It should not be taken that I subscribe to the James-Lange theory of the emotions, based on the views of William James (1884), where physiological arousal is seen as an essential component of emotion states and which then implies a universal basis to the emotions. I find it more useful to follow Solomon, who defines an emotion as 'a system of concepts, beliefs, attitudes and desires, virtually all of which are context-bound, historically

developed, and culture specific' (1984: 249). While this does not rule out a physiological element, it throws the emphasis onto the cultural interpretation, so that the type of overlap that then exists between such concepts cross-culturally becomes a matter for ethnographic inquiry. However, of interest for the Gisu concepts is Solomon's speculation that 'a culture that emphasises what David Hume called 'the violent passions' will be ripe for the Jamesian theory, but a culture that rather stresses the 'calm' emotions (an appreciation of beauty, lifelong friendship, a sense of beneficence and justice) will find the Jamesian theory and the hydraulic model that underlies it patently absurd' (1984: 242).

2 The rate quoted here is calculated from police figures and is the average for the ten-year period, 1945–54. It is thus comparable to the rate quoted for 1963, again calculated from police figures by R.E. Turner and cited in Belshaw et al. (1966). My own figures, calculated from the Death Enquiry Reports filed by the Police in the District Court, give a slightly higher average annual homicide rate of thirty-two deaths per 100,000 for the years between 1960 and 1966. The percentage figures given are calculated from the court case records for this period (see Heald 1998).

3 Some caution needs to be exercised with this interpretation since much of it rests on Spencer's understanding of the trembling and shaking of the *moran* as nervous behaviour evidencing anxiety and even 'transmarginal' breakdown. This raises the whole question of our ability to recognise and identify emotions from behavioural symptoms alone, a relevant query when Spencer later tells us that the *moran* link shaking with anger. Given the association in Kenya of shaking with warriorhood – as generally signalling a readiness to fight – it is a pity that further consideration of Samburu concepts was omitted from the discussion. This is not of course to deny the relevance of some form of operant conditioning for an understanding of the psychological processes involved in Samburu rituals.

4 Where this is not the case, and values are apparently at variance, then the psychological effects are often difficult to establish, as the controversy over television violence illustrates, with both cathartic and disinhibitionary effects receiving support from experimental studies (Geen et al., 1975; Kaplan and Singer, 1976; Konecni and Ebbersen, 1976).

5 I am grateful to Terezia Hinga for pointing out to me the similarity between the Kikuyu and Gisu concepts.

4 EVERY MAN A HERO: OEDIPAL THEMES IN
GISU CIRCUMCISION

1 I am indebted to Reg Hook for helping to clarify a number of issues in this paper in the stimulating discussions we had in Canberra in 1991, and to Florence Bégoin-Guinard and Vincent Crapanzano for their perceptive comments on this paper during and after the colloquium on *Culture, Psychanalyse, Interprétation*, held in Paris in July 1991.

2 While the phylogenetic implications of Freud's *Totem and Taboo* have usually been dropped in favour of the ontogenetic, this line of argument, though with variations as to stress, is to be found in the earlier work of Roheim (e.g., 1934), Whiting et al. (1958) and more recently in Spiro (1982), Ottenberg (1988).

3 See especially, Fortes, 1966, 1977 and Turner, 1967.
4 Though, at the same time, it is possible to see it as an occasion when men are able to display their complementary Oedipal aggression (see Spiro, 1982) in both their taunts and their identification with individual candidates.
5 This prohibition is given its greatest expression in the avoidance relationships of a man with his mother-in-law and daughter-in-law. This relationship, as I have described, serves as a prototype for all forbidden sexual relationships. See Chapter Seven of this volume.
6 Their area of competition is that of the 'penis' (*ihando*), the word used of heritable property. By contrast the property exchanges that accompany marriage are referred to as *buxwe*, a term which is also used of sexual shame.
7 Personal communication.
8 One can note, however, that the phallic-shaped ends of banana bunches are, in some areas, thrown onto the roof of the house as the boy stands for the operation in his father's compound. Again, I never heard this interpreted, but the message again might be that of the 'flowering'.

5 WITCHES AND THIEVES: DEVIANT MOTIVATIONS IN GISU SOCIETY

I am grateful to Ivan Karp and David Parkin for their comments on an earlier draft of this chapter.

1 In Kenya this pattern is reported not only for the Kikuyu but for the Kamba (Middleton and Kershaw, 1965) and the Babukusu (Wagner, 1940).
2 A similar bias is apparent in the historical study of European witchcraft which scholars have treated as a *crimen exceptum*, removing it from the general context of crime and social control in so doing. Witchcraft, the 'impossible crime', is deemed to require a specific and distinct explanation. Larner (1984) points out that this is due to present-day cultural bias as much as to the factors that made it a *crimen exceptum* with regard to the difficulty of establishing guilt in the sixteenth and seventeenth centuries.
3 For more detail see Heald, 1986, 1998.
4 Women generally are marginal to Gisu homicide patterns, which overwhelmingly comprise cases where men kill men.
5 The small number of witch-killings reflects a low rate of prosecution in such cases.
6 These rates were calculated from the Death Enquiry Reports filed at the Court by the Police on the basis of their first investigation into cases of suspicious death for the years between 1964 and 1968.
7 For example, Becker 1963; Cohen 1971; Goffman 1968.

6 DIVINATORY FAILURE: GISU DIVINERS AND THE PROBLEM OF DOUBT

I am very grateful to Vernon Pratt and to the editors of the journal *Africa* issue 61(3) for their helpful comments on an earlier draft of this chapter.

1 The exact frequency is hard to establish, partly because of the difficulty of deciding who is to count as a diviner in a situation where many people are 'caught', practise for a while, then let it fall away, while others never practise at all. In this situation all that it is safe to say is that almost everyone would have a practising diviner operating within a few hundred yards of their homestead. There is little clustering of specialists, as is the case in some other areas of East Africa. For example, among the Giriama, in one area, out of fifty-four homes thirty-seven had knowledge of medicines, eighteen were diviners, eleven were sorcery cleansers, fourteen were specialists of other kinds and eight were sorcerers (Thompson, 1990). This was an unusual area, a focal point of both good and evil possessory spirits, but it is interesting in giving a clear indication of just how common such specialists may be.

2 Gisu divination bears a close resemblance to that of their Nyole neighbours; Whyte (1988) also takes up this issue and the indeterminacy of the divinatory process.

3 Horton (1967) in fact does not argue this, since, although he is concerned to demonstrate affinities between the structure of traditional thought and modern science, he concludes that major differences can be attributed to the intellectual closure of traditional thought as against the 'open' nature of Western thought. Further, while this contrast is applied at the level of the belief systems and not supposedly to individual attitudes and responses it in fact tends to spill over and colour these too. In expanding upon the propositions of closure, he writes of a magical attitude to words, of a belief system which is protected at all costs by taboo and secondary elaboration, and of the anxiety that any challenge to existing tenets arouses. Again the situational groundedness of knowledge is seen to work against the critical faculties. Thus, despite the radicalness of Horton's attempt to break down the old dichotomies between modern and traditional thought, ultimately we are left again with the picture of the hidebound traditional thinker completely committed to the terms of his belief.

4 See also the interesting discussion in Marwick (1973) in which he argues that our lack of knowledge and control in the modern West breeds not the 'open society' envisaged by Popper but a pervasive cynical scepticism.

5 This is as evident in the classroom as in the consulting room, where children are taught that different contexts each imply their own forms of knowledge and 'trust'; the acceptance of information given by the teacher, even where it runs counter to accepted and known practice, has been identified as a key element in pupil 'success' (Keddie, 1971).

6 The work of Cole et al. (1971) is relevant here. In talking about the refusal of nonliterate Kpelle of West Africa to accept the logical task implied by verbal syllogism, they found that the Kpelle tended to be guided by their knowledge, by what they knew to be the case, rather than by the logic of the puzzle itself. Their responses implied a definite refusal to take knowledge imparted by the investigator on trust, to accept a hypothetical situation as against their own past experience.

7 Reviewing the literature on the psychological factors in clinical trials, Gilmour (1977) deals with the importance of the doctor/patient relationship and how the placebo effects are affected by the doctor's enthusiasm for a new drug. He comments that 'It is a commonly observed phenomenon

that there is a gradual decline in the effectiveness of new treatments after the first flush of enthusiasm for them has worn off' (1977: 157).

8 My views on Gisu divination are deeply coloured by the fact that few of the situations which led to divination that I witnessed could be said to have had a happy outcome. In part this is due to the fact mentioned that the Gisu do not resort to divination except in situations of acute illness or persistent misfortune. Cure was rare and remission short-lived.

9 For example, Evans-Pritchard (1940) and Rigby (1975). Rigby argues that among the Ganda the same individual may be able to shift to and fro between the role of diviner and prophet.

7 JOKING AND AVOIDANCE, HOSTILITY AND INCEST: AN ESSAY ON GISU MORAL CATEGORIES

I am very grateful to Ray Abrahams, Mary Douglas, Tim Ingold, Ivan Karp, Anne Sharman and Jean Smith for their comments on an earlier version of this article and for the constructive discussion offered during the ESRC workshop 'Accounts of human nature' held in Windsor in March 1988.

1 For further details, see Heald (1998).

2 From this point of view there are only two generations, with adjacent generations reproducing each other while alternate generations replicate each other. Thus, physical substance is transmitted between the generations from parents to children while 'life force' is inherited from grandparents to grandchildren. A person is named after the person whose life force he is deemed to have inherited and, most commonly, this is from someone who has recently died in the grandparental generation.

3 The cousins excluded by these arrangements are the mother's sister's children who, significantly, are known as *bamusoni* (sing. *umusoni*) and with whom the relationship approaches avoidance. One of the worst forms of incest is that with an *umusoni* and the term, from the same root as *tsisoni*, implies the sexually forbidden. Variations of the term are used elsewhere in the kinship terminology. Thus, relatives of the third ascending or descending generation are known by the reciprocal term *cisoni* (pl. *bisoni*). In all cases where these terms are used a magnification of sexual restriction is implied, and possibly an emphatic restatement of a principle. For example, the third ascending and descending generations represent the limits of absolute marriage prohibition since it is usually considered possible to marry those related from the fourth generation. See also note 5.

4 *Basoni* is not strictly speaking a kinship term as it is not usually used either in address or reference. Its usage rather is descriptive. Such relatives, alternatively, may be described as *baxwe*; derived from the root, *xwa*, to marry, through the exchange of bridewealth, *buxwe*. Again, this carries the connotation of sexual prohibition.

5 In rare cases a man may inherit a widow from the senior generation, but only in the event that he was already adult at the time of the initial marriage so that she could never have acted as a 'mother' to him.

6 This series does not include all kinship relationships, but one can note that in the Gisu system the relationship with the mother's brother, although

terminologically distinct, is akin to that with the father with whom he is closely identified by virtue of being his 'brother-in-law' and man of the senior generation. The relationship is one of restraint. Likewise, the relationship with the father's sister is likened to that with the mother.

7 The relationship between brothers and sisters is characterised by affection and their equality is often marked by the use of the term *yaya*, 'comrade', to address each other. For a man to address his wife as 'sister' is a mark both of esteem and affection.

8 Stephens and D'Andrade (1962) have noted a strong empirical association of extreme kin avoidance with licentious joking patterns, to the extent of suggesting that the world may be divided up between 'avoiding' and 'non-avoiding' societies. Their hypothesis that such avoidances represent a phobic reaction to incest motivated by Oedipal conflicts is consistent with the interpretation of mother-in-law avoidance later advanced in this chapter. This line of causality, however, runs against the emphasis here on the symbolic construction of the kinship universe in terms of a patterning of permissible behaviours. Indeed, as they admit, while the postulate of Oedipal conflict might 'explain' mother-in-law avoidance in terms of a displacement of desire, it fails to account for the joking relationship or, indeed, for the association between the two forms.

9 *Bamasaala* has more limited reference than the other terms (*basoni* and *baxwe*) used of people of the opposite sex and generation. It is used only of WM/DH and HF/SW, though, since it includes all relatives in these categories (e.g., all women whom the wife addresses as 'mother') of oneself and close relatives, it is in fact subject to wide extension. It derives from the root, *saala*, to give birth or beget.

10 Parkin (1986) has contrasted 'raw fear' of this and with 'respectful fear', with the latter seen as an instrument of hierarchy and calculable in its consequences in a way that the former is not.

11 Gisu marriage rules permit only a one-way flow of women. A marriage may thus initiate a series of marriages in the same direction but there can be no sister exchange nor any other form of exchange marriage.

12 I have discussed elsewhere (Heald, 1998) this theme of peacemaking in the context of East African societies, where the idea that 'joking relationships' originate from a prior state of hostility is widespread. The Gisu present the greatest elaboration upon this symbolic theme and the evidence points to the fact that it was the main mechanism for finishing feuds among neighbouring lineages in the past. The structural context for this unique form of peace-pact appears to be that of small, relatively weak kinship groups living in close proximity and linked by marriage and matri-filiation. See also Tew (1953).

13 Kuper (1982b) has developed a sophisticated interpretation of this and of joking among affines, relating its forms to bridewealth exchanges among the peoples of southern Africa.

14 Thus, as Howell (1973) puts it, the 'exercise and acceptance of licence' may be used to mark and test a relationship, but the element of risk makes it inappropriate in really close, intimate relationships. Yet, the absence of teasing forms here poses evident problems for Howell's thesis with its emphasis on solidarity, a problem which he solves by proposing that it is potential intimacy, a 'willingness to be close' which is symbolised.

Potential closeness, however, seems predicated upon the fact of separation, leading one to conclude that if the thrust of Howell's argument runs counter to that of Radcliffe-Brown, the substance remains remarkably unchanged.

8   THE POWER OF SEX: REFLECTIONS ON THE CALDWELLS' 'AFRICAN SEXUALITY' THESIS

1 The latter two authors have both been concerned to show that among the Kikuyu (Ahlberg) and Meru (Chege), traditional sexual practices had a decidedly puritanical edge. Both also argue that Christianity, far from encouraging a greater moral value being attached to sexual intercourse, in practice, because of its attack on the indigenous moral system in conjunction with Colonial administrative and economic changes, it operated to loosen customary controls around sexuality.

2 For a useful overview of this issue, see Kuper, 1982a.

3 In other societies such privileged access extended not to lineage brothers but to other key relationships such as age mates, as among the Kuria of south-west Kenya.

4 The degree to which such 'privileged access' was allowable and the circumstances that facilitated it require in-depth examination of particular societies. It seems that it was much more likely to be invoked in situations where the husband was absent, for example, for prolonged periods of labour migration or, in cases, of impotence. It thus seems likely that its use has grown since colonisation.

5 While I describe the Gisu system in the ethnographic present, this fieldwork was done between 1965 and 1969 and thus reports patterns current some twenty-five years ago. I have no knowledge of the changes that may have taken place in Bugisu in the interim war-torn conditions that have characterised Uganda. Current research among the Kuria of rural Kenya, however, despite considerable change, points to the continuing strength of traditional belief and of the rules of respect.

6 For more details on Gisu kinship etiquette, kinship and the concepts of respect and avoidance, see Chapter Seven of this volume.

7 See Heald, 1998, and Chapters Two, Three and Four of this volume.

8 Kenyatta, 1938; Chege, 1993; Ahlberg, 1994.

9 As the Caldwells (1989) point out the evidence contained in this book is often unclear and complicated in some instances by different anthropologists giving contradictory views. In some societies, pre-marital pregnancy attracted sanctions (often extremely severe ones) but the question of absolute chastity was less of an issue. However, if one simply takes the evidence on the desirability of virginity of girls at marriage, one finds that out of twenty-eight societies described in the volume, in eleven, virginity was said to be an important prerequisite for girls in the past and often also at the present. By contrast, for only seven societies did the ethnographers report that no value at all was set on virginity. The other ten cases were indeterminate, either because no information was provided on the issue or the writing was ambiguous. The implications of chastity rules for the status of women are well discussed by Southall, 1960b.

10 Another well-known case in point is the *ngweko* practice of the neigh-bouring Kikuyu first described by Kenyatta, 1938. Here the circumcised youth were allowed considerable freedom in both courtship and sex play but full intercourse was forbidden and prevented by the girls firmly tying their leather skirts and aprons between their thighs.

11 See Parkin, 1973; Potash, 1978; Obbo, 1976.

12 See Heald 1998 and Chapters Two and Seven of this volume.

13 See further, Chapter Four of this volume.

14 See Beidelman, 1986, Richards, 1956a; Wilson, 1957; Berglund, 1976; Ngubane, 1976 and for further comments on fire and sexuality, Ruel, 1985.

15 This should not be imagined as some kind of collective orgy. The darkness of the night simply allowed couples to slip away with no questions asked.

9   TRIBAL RITES AND TRIBAL RIGHTS

I am most grateful to Fred Klaits, Mike Neocosmos, Doo Selolwane and Daniel Nsereko for giving their time to reading and commenting upon drafts of this chapter. My thanks also go to Joseph Maroa Mwita and Wekesa Wekola for their ethnographic acumen.

1 I am grateful to David Mills for first bringing this case to my attention and to Daniel Nsereko for the information on the religious convictions of this family. In fact, Kabala's father was a pastor in a SDA church. The SDA belief in the body as the Temple of the Lord puts particular emphasis on the healthy, immaculate body and the avoidance of contamination. It is thus no coincidence that in areas of Kenya, such as Kuria District, where girls are clitoridectomised, it is as yet only the SDAs, and only a few of those families, who have eschewed the operation. In Kuria, however, they have not opposed the circumcision of boys.

2 The January issue of *The New Vision* mentions that there had not been a case of a forced circumcision being prosecuted since colonial days.

3 It is worth highlighting the unusualness of this in the East African context. I know of no other Ugandan or Kenya society where transsexualism of this kind is mentioned in the literature and Kenyan friends insist that it is unknown.

4 According to the *Weekly Review* of 19 July 1991, seventy girls were raped and nineteen died. According to some other newspaper reports of the time, rape seemed hardly to amount to an offence at all in the eyes of local people. People around the school made no attempt to intervene, some explaining that they heard the girls crying and screaming many Saturday nights and 'it was usually just because the boys were trying to rape them'.

5 Among the Kuria, for example, coitus is regarded as gratifying only for men and female pleasure is conventionally assumed to be absent. While the Kuria practice clitoridectomy and the Gisu do not, it would over-simplify this issue to relate it only to the presence or absence of such operations.

BIBLIOGRAPHY

Abrahams, R.D. and Bauman, R. (1978) 'Ranges of festival behavior', in
B. Babcock (ed.) *The Reversible World*, Ithaca, NJ: Cornell University Press.
Ahern, E. (1979) 'The problem of efficacy: strong and weak illocutionary acts',
Man n.s 14: 1–17.
Ahlberg, B.M. (1994) 'Is there a distinct African sexuality? A critical response
to Caldwell *et al.*', *Africa* 64: 220–42.
Anderson, B. (1983) *Imagined Communities: Reflections on the Origin and Spread
of Nationalism*. London: Verso.
Apthorpe, R. (1967) 'Nsenga social ideas.' *Mawazo* 1: 23–30.
Beattie, J. (1966) 'Ritual and Social Change.' *Man n.s.* 1: 60–74.
—— (1970) 'On Understanding Ritual', in B. Wilson (ed.) *Rationality*, Oxford:
Basil Blackwell.
Becker, H.S. (1963) *Outsiders*. New York: Collier-Macmillan.
Beidelman, T.O. (1966) 'Utani – some Kaguru notions of death, sexuality and
affinity.' *Southwestern Journal of Anthropropology* 22: 354–81.
—— (1986) *Moral Imagination in Kaguru Models of Thought*. Bloomington, IA:
Indiana University Press.
Belshaw, D.G., Brock, B. and Wallace, I. (1966) *The Bugisu Coffee Industry: an
Economic and Technical Survey*. Report for the International Bank for
Reconstruction and Development.
Berglund, A.L. (1976) *Zulu Thought Patterns and Symbolism*. London: Hurst.
Bergson, H. (1921) *Laughter: An Essay on the Meaning of the Comic*. London:
Macmillan.
Bettelheim, B. (1954) *Symbolic Wounds*. Glencoe, IL: The Free Press.
Bitek, O. p' (1973) *Africa's Cultural Revolution*. Nairobi: Macmillan.
Brod, H (ed.) (1987) *The Making of Masculinities: New Men's Studies*. Winch-
ester, MA: Allen and Unwin.
Burke, K. (1945) *A Grammar of Motives*. Englewood Cliffs, NJ: Prentice-Hall.
Caldwell, J. C. and Caldwell, P. (1987) 'The cultural context of high fertility
in Sub-Saharan Africa'. *Population and Development Review* 13: 409–37.
Caldwell, J. C., Caldwell, P. and Quiggin, (1989) 'The social context of AIDS
in Sub-Saharan Africa', *Population and Development Review*, 15: 185–234.

Caldwell, J. C., Orubulwe, I. and Caldwell, P. (1991) 'The Destablilisation of the Traditional Yoruba Sexual System'. *Population and Development Review* 17: 229–62.

Carrigan, T, Connell, B. and Lee, J. (1987) 'Towards a New Sociology of Masculinity'. In H. Brod (ed.) *The Making of Masculinities: New Men's Studies*. Winchester, MA: Allen and Unwin.

Chanock, M. (1985) *Law, Custom and Social Order: The Colonial Experience in Malawi and Zambia*. Cambridge: Cambridge University Press.

Chege, J. (1993) 'The Politics of Gender and Fertility Regulation in Kenya: A case study of the Igembe', unpublished PhD thesis, Lancaster University.

Cohen, P. (1980) 'Psychoanalysis and Cultural Symbolization', in M.L. Foster and S.H. Brandes (eds) *Symbol as Sense*. London: Academic Press.

Cohen, S. (ed.) (1971) *Images of Deviance*. Harmondsworth: Penguin.

Cohen, D. and Odhiambo, E. (1992) *Burying SM: The Politics of Knowledge and the Sociology of Power in Africa*. London: James Currey.

Cole, M., Gay, J., Glick, J. and Sharp, D. (1971) *The Cultural Context of Learning and Thinking*. London: Methuen.

Comaroff, J. (1985) *Body of Power, Spirit of Resistance*. Chicago: University of Chicago Press.

Connell, R.W. (1995) *Masculinities*. Oxford: Polity Press.

Cornwall, A. and Lindisfarne, N. (eds) (1994) *Dislocating Masculinity: Comparative Ethnographies*. London: Routledge.

Crick, M. (1976) *Explorations in Language and Meaning*. London: Malaby Press.

Devereux, G. (1961) 'Art and Mythology: a general theory', in B. Kaplan (ed.) *Studying Personality Cross-Culturally*. Illinois: Row, Peterson and Comp.

Douglas, M. (1966) *Purity and Danger: An Analysis of Concepts of Pollution and Taboo*. London: Routledge & Kegan Paul.

—— (1968) 'The social control of cognition: some factors in joke perception', *Man* n.s 3: 3610–76.

—— (1982) 'The effects of modernisation on religious change'. *Daedelas* 3:1–19.

Durkheim, E. (1961) *The Elementary Forms of the Religious Life*. London: Collier Books edition.

Evans-Pritchard, E. E. (1933) 'Zande blood brotherhood'. *Africa* 6: 369–401.

—— (1937) *Witchcraft, Oracles and Magic among the Azande*. Oxford: Clarendon Press.

—— (1940) *The Nuer*. Oxford: Clarendon Press.

—— (1951) *Kinship and Marriage among the Nuer*. Oxford: Clarendon Press.

Fadiman, J.A. (1982) *An Oral History of Tribal Warfare: The Meru of Mt. Kenya*. Ohio: Ohio University Press.

Feierman, S. (1990) *Peasant Intellectuals. Anthropology and History in Tanzania*. Madison: University of Wisconsin Press.

Fortes, M. (1966) 'Totem and Taboo'. *Proceedings of the Royal Anthropological Institute* 5–22.

—— (1977) 'Custom and Conscience in Anthropological Perspective'. *International Review of Psychoanalysis* 4:127–54.

Freedman, S. (1977) 'Joking, affinity and the exchange of ritual services among the Kiga of Northern Ruanda: an essay on joking relationship theory'. *Man* n.s. 12: 154–65.

Freud, S. (1950) *Totem and Taboo*. London: Routledge & Kegan Paul.

—— (1951) *Moses and Monotheism*. London: The Hogarth Press.

—— (1960) *Jokes and Their Relation to the Unconscious*. London: Routledge & Kegan Paul.

Garfinkel, H. (1956) 'The conditions of successful degradation ceremonies'. *American Journal of Sociology* 61: 240–44.

Geen, R.G. *et al.*(1975) 'The facilitation of aggression by aggression: evidence against the catharsis hypothesis'. *Journal of Personality and Social Psychology* 31(4): 721–6.

Geertz, C. (1957) 'Ritual and social change: A Javanese Example'. *American Anthropologist* 59: 32–54.

—— (1966) 'Religion as a Cultural System', in M. Banton (ed.) *Anthropological Approaches to the Study of Religion*. London: Tavistock.

—— (1973) 'Person, time and conduct in Bali', in *The Interpretation of Cultures*. New York: Basic Books.

—— (1983) 'From the native's point of view: on the nature of anthropological understanding' in *Local Knowledge: Further Essays in Interpretive Anthropology*, New York: Basic Books.

Gennep, A. Van. (1960) *The Rites of Passage*. London: Routledge & Kegan Paul.

Gilmour, R. (1977) 'Psychological factors in clinical trials', in S.N. Johnson and S. Johnson (eds.), *Clinical Trials*. Oxford: Blackwell.

Girard, R. (1977) *Violence and the Sacred*. Baltimore and London: Johns Hopkins University Press.

Gluckman, M. (1963) *Order and Rebellion in Tribal Africa*. London: Cohen.

—— (ed.) (1964) *Closed Systems and Open Minds: the limits of Naiveté in Social Anthropology*. Edinburgh and London: Oliver and Boyd.

Golfman, E. (1968) *Stigma: notes on the management of spoiled identity*. Harmondsworth: Penguin.

Goody, J. (1961) 'Religion and ritual: The definitional problem'. *British Journal of Sociology* 12: 142–63.

Goody, J. and Watt, I. (1968) 'The consequences of literacy', in J. Goody (ed.) *Literacy in Traditional Societies*. Cambridge: Cambridge University Press.

Hall, S. (1996) 'Introduction: Who Needs 'Identity'?', in S. Hall and P. du Gay (eds) *Questions of Cultural Identity*. London: Sage.

Handelman, D. (1982) 'Reflexivity in festivals and other cultural events', in M. Douglas (ed.) *Essays in the Sociology of Perception*. London: Roudedge & Kegan Paul.

Hawkins, R. and Heald, S. (1988) *Imbalu: Ritual of Manhood of the Gisu of Uganda*. Videotape distributed by the Royal Anthropological Institute.

Heald, S. (1986) 'Mafias in Africa: the rise of drinking companies and vigilante groups in Bugisu District, Uganda', *Africa* 56(4): 446–67.

—— (1998) [1989] *Controlling Anger: The Anthropology of Gisu Violence.* London: James Currey. First published by Manchester University Press.

Heider, F. (1958) *The Psychology of Interpersonal Relations.* New York: Wiley.

—— and Deluz, A. (eds) (1994) *Anthropology and Psychoanalysis: An Encounter Through Culture.* London and New York: Routledge.

Herdt, G. H. (1982) *Rituals of Manhood: Male Initiations in Papua New Guinea.* Berkeley, LA and London: University of California Press.

Hiatt, L.R. (1971) 'Secret Pseudo-procreative rites among the Australian Aborigines', in L.R. Hiatt and C. Jayawardena (eds) *Anthropology in Oceania.* San Francisco: Chandler.

Hiatt, L.R. (1975) 'Introduction' to L.R. Hiatt (ed.) *Australian Aboriginal Mythology.* Canberra: Australian Institute for Aboriginal Studies.

Hobsbawn, E. and Ranger, T. (eds) (1983) *The Invention of Tradition.* Cambridge: Cambridge University Press.

Homans, G. (1941) 'Anxiety and ritual: the theories of Malinowski and Radcliffe-Brown'. *American Anthropologist* 43:164–72.

Horton, R. (1960) 'A definition of religion and its uses'. *Journal of the Royal Anthropological Institute* 90: 201–26.

—— (1967) 'African traditional thought and Western science'. *Africa* 37(1,2): 50–71; 155–87.

Howell, R.W. (1973) 'Teasing relationships'. *Addison-Wesley Module Anthrop.* 46.

Howell, S. (1997) *The Ethnography of Moralities.* London: Routledge.

Jackson, M. (1978) 'An approach to Kuranko divination'. *Human Relations* 31(1): 117–38.

James, Wendy (1988) *The Listening Ebony: Moral Knowledge, Religion and Power among the Uduk of the Sudan.* Oxford: Clarendon Press.

James, William (1984) 'What is an emotion?' *Mind* 9:188–205.

Jones, E.E. and Nisbett, R.E. (1971) *The Actor and the Observer: Divergent Perceptions of the Causes of Behaviour.* New Jersey: General Learning Press.

Kapferer, B. (1979) 'Mind, self and other in demonic illness: the negation and reconstruction of self'. *American Ethnologist* 6: 110–33.

Kaplan, R. M. and Singer, R. D. (1976) 'Television violence and viewer aggression: a re-examination of the evidence'. *Journal of Social Issues* 32: 18–34.

Karp, I. and Karp, P. (1973) 'The Iteso of Kenya', in A. Molnos (ed.) *Cultural Source Materials for Population Planning in East Africa III: Beliefs and Practices.* Nairobi: University of Nairobi.

Keddie, N. (1971) 'Classroom knowledge'. in M. Young (ed.), *Knowledge and Control.* London: Collier-Macmillan.

Kelly, H.H. (1971) *Attribution in Social Interaction.* London: Secker and Warburg.

Kennedy, J. G. (1970) 'Bonds of laughter among the Tarahumara Indians: towards the rethinking of joking relationship theory', in W. Goldschmidt and H. Hoijer (eds) *The social anthropology of Latin America.* Berkeley, LA: University of California Latin American Studies Center.

Kenyatta, J. (1938) *Facing Mount Kenya.* London: Secker and Warburg.

Kisekka, M.N. (1973) 'Baganda of Central Uganda', in A. Molnos (ed.) *Cultural Source materials for population planning in East Africa. vol 111: Beliefs and Practices.* Institute of African Studies, University of Nairobi.

Klein, M. (1989) *The Oedipus complex in the light of early anxieties.* (originally 1945) Reprinted in R. Britton *et al., The Oedipus Complex Today.* London: Karnac Books.

Koestler, A. (1964) *The Act of Creation.* London: Picador.

Konecni, V.J. and Ebbersen, E.B. (1976) 'Disinhibition versus the Cathartic effect: artifact and substance'. *Journal of Personality and Social Psychology* 34(3): 352–65.

Kuper, A. (1982a) 'Lineage theory: A critical retrospect'. *Annual Review of Anthropology* 11:71–95.

—— (1982b) *Cattle for wives.* London: Routledge & Kegan Paul.

La Fontaine, J.S. (1957) 'The Social Organisation of the Gisu of Uganda with Special Reference to their initiation ceremonies', unpublished PhD thesis, Cambridge University.

—— (1959) *The Gisu of Uganda.* Ethnographic Survey of Africa, London: International Afncan Institute.

—— (1960) 'Homicide and suicide among the Gisu, in P. Bohannan (ed.) *African Homicide and Suicide.* Princeton, NJ: Princeton University Press.

—— (1963) 'Witchcraft in Bugisu', in J. Middleton and E.H. Winter (eds) *Witchcraft and Sorcery in East Africa.* London: Routledge & Kegan Paul.

—— (1967) 'Parricide in Bugisu: a study in intergenerational conflict'. *Man* n.s. 2: 249–59.

—— (1969) 'Tribalism among the Gisu', in P. H. Gulliver (ed.) *Tradition and Transition in East Africa.* London: Routledge & Kegan Paul.

—— (1971) 'Ritualisation of women's life crises in Bugisu', in *The Interpretation of Ritual.* London: Tavistock.

—— (1977) 'The power of rights'. *Man* n.s. 12: 421–37.

Lacan, J. (1977) *Ecrits: A Selection.* London:Tavistock.

Lambert, H. E. (1912–18) *Disintegration and Reintegration in the Meru Tribe.* Kenya National Archives 1912–18.

Lan, D. (1985) *Guns and Rain: guerrillas and spirit mediums in Zimbabwe.* London: James Currey.

Larner, C. (1984) *Witchcraft and Religion: The politics of Popular Belief.* Oxford: Basil Blackwell.

Le Blanc, M.N., Meintel, D. and Piche, V. (1991) 'The African sexual system: comments on Caldwell *et al.*'. *Population and Development Review* 1 (3): 497–505.

Leach, E. R. (1958) 'Magical Hair', *Journal of the Royal Anthropological Institute,* 88(2): 147–64.

Lemaire, A. (1977) *Jacques Lacan.* London: Routledge & Kegan Paul.

Lévi-Strauss, C. (1966) *The Savage Mind*. London: Weidenfeld & Nicolson.

LeVine, R.A. (1959) 'Gusii sex offences: A study of social control'. *American Anthropologist* 61: 965–90.

—— (1984) 'Properties of culture: an ethnographic view', in R.A. Shweder and R.A. LeVine (eds) *Culture Theory: Essays on mind, self, and emotion*. Cambridge: Cambridge University Press.

Lewis, I.M. (1966) 'Spirit possession and deprivation cults', *Man n.s.*, 1 (3): 307–29.

—— (1971) *Ecstatic Religion: An Anthropological Study of Spirit Possession and Shamanism*. London: Penguin.

Lidz, R.W. and Lidz, T. (1977) 'Male menstruation: A ritual alternative to Oedipal transition'. *International Journal of Psychoanalysis* 58: 17–31.

—— (1984) 'Oedipus in the Stone Age'. *Journal of the American Psychoanalytic Association* 32 (3): 507–28.

Lonsdale, J. (1992) 'The moral economy of Mau Mau: The problem', in B. Berman and J. Lonsdale, *Unhappy Valley: Conflict in Kenya and Africa*. Book 2. London: James Currey.

Malinowski, B. (1926) *Crime and Custom in Savage Society*. London: Kegan Paul.

—— (1945) *Magic, Science and Religion*. Glencoe, IL: The Free Press.

Marwick, M. (1965) *Sorcery in its Social Setting*. Manchester: Manchester University Press.

—— (1973) 'How real is the charmed circle in African and Western thought?' *Africa* 43(1): 59–70.

Mauss, M. (1972) *A General Theory of Magic*. London: Routledge & Kegan Paul.

Middleton, J. (1960) *Lugbara Religion*. London: Oxford University Press.

Middleton, J. and Kershaw, G. (1965) *The Kikuyu and Kamba of Kenya*. London: Oxford University Press for the International African Institute.

Middleton, J. and Winter, E.H. (eds) (1963) *Witchcraft and Sorcery in East Africa*. London: Routledge & Kegan Paul.

Mitchell, J.C. (1956) *The Yao Village*. Manchester: Manchester University Press.

Molnos, A. (1973) *Cultural Source materials for population planning in East Africa. vol 3: Beliefs and Practices*. Institute of African Studies, University of Nairobi.

Moore, S.F. (1975) 'Selection for failure in a small social field: Ritual concord and fraternal strife among the Chagga, Kilimanjaro, 1968–1969', in S.F. Moore and B. Myerhoff (eds) *Symbol and Politics in Communal Ideology*. Ithaca, NY: Cornell University Press.

Morton, J. (1990) 'Introduction: Geza Roheim's contribution to Australian ethnography', in J. Morton and W. Muensterberger (eds) *Children of the Desert 11*. Oceania Ethnographies 2, Sydney: University of Sydney Press.

Ngubane, H. (1976) 'Some notions of "purity" and "impurity" among the Zulu'. *Africa* 46 (3): 274–84.

Obbo, C. (1976) 'Dominant male ideology and female options: Three East Africa Case Studies'. *Africa* 46(4) 371–88.

Ocaya-Lakidi, Dent, (1979) 'Manhood, warriorhood and sex in Eastern Africa'. *Journal of Asian and African Studies* 134–65.

Ottenberg, S. (1988) 'Oedipus, gender and social solidarity: A case study of male childhood and initiation'. *Ethos* 16: 326–52.

Park, G. (1963) 'Divination and its social contexts'. *Journal of the Royal Anthropological Institute* 93(2): 195–219.

Parkin, D. (1968) 'Medicines and men of influence'. *Man n.s.* 3(3): 424–39.

—— (1973) 'Luo of Kampala, Nairobi and Western Kenya', in A. Molnos (ed.) *Cultural Source materials for population planning in East Africa. vol 111.* Institute of African Studies, University of Nairobi.

—— (1986) 'Towards an apprehension of Fear', in D.L. Scuton (ed.) *Sociophobics: the anthropology of fear.* Boulder, London: Westview Press.

Peel, J.D.Y. (1969) 'Understanding alien belief systems'. *British Journal of Sociology* 20: 69–84.

Perryman, P.W. (1937) 'Native witchcraft'. *Uganda Journal* 4(1): 7–27.

Polanyi, M. and Prosch, H. (1975) *Meaning.* Chicago: University of Chicago Press.

Popper, K. (1945) *The Open Society and its Enemies.* London: Routledge.

Potash, B. (1978) 'Some aspects of marital stability in a rural Luo community'. *Africa* 48 (4): 380–96.

Purvis, Rev. J.B. (1909) *Through Uganda to Mount Elgon.* London: T. Fisher Unwin.

Radcliffe-Brown, A.R. (1924) 'The mother's brother in South Africa'. *South African Journal of Social Science* 21: 542–55.

—— (1940) 'On joking relationships', *Africa* 13, 195–210.

—— (1940) 'Preface' to E.E. Evans-Pritchard and M. Fortes (eds) *African Political Systems.* Oxford: Oxford University Press.

—— (1949) 'A further note on joking relationships', *Africa* 19, 133–40.

—— (1952) *Structure and Function in Primitive Society,* Glencoe, Ill: The Free Press.

Ranger, T. (1993) 'The invention of tradition revisited: The case of colonial Africa'. In T. Ranger and O. Vaughan (eds) *Legitimacy and the State in Twentieth Century Africa.* London: Macmillan.

Raum, O.F. (1973) 'Chaga of North-eastern Tanzania', in A. Molnos (ed.) *Cultural Source materials for population planning in East Africa. vol 3: Beliefs and Practices.* Institute of African Studies, University of Nairobi.

Read, K.E. (1955) 'Morality and the concept of the person among the Gahuku-Gama'. *Oceania* XXV(4): 233–82.

Reik, T. (1931) *Ritual.* London: Hogarth Press.

Richards, A. I. (1937) 'Reciprocal clan relationships among the Bemba'. *Man n.s.* 2: 22.

—— (1956a) *Chisungu: A Girls' Initiation Ceremony Among the Bemba of Northern Rhodesia.* London: Faber & Faber.

—— (1956b) *Economic Development and Tribal Change*. Cambridge: Heffer.

—— (1967) 'African Systems of Thought: an Anglo-French dialogue' (review article). *Man n.s.* 2: 286–98.

—— (1970) 'Socialisation and contemporary British anthropology', in P. Mayer (ed.) *Socialisation: The Approach frown Social Anthropology*. London: Tavistock Press.

Richards, I. A. (1936) *Philosophy of Rhetoric*. Oxford: Oxford University Press.

Ricoeur, P. (1979) 'Psychoanalysis and the movement of contemporary culture', in P. Rabinow and W.M. Sullivan (eds) *Interpretive Social Science: A Reader*. Berkeley, LA: University of California Press.

—— (1981) 'The question of proof in Freud's psychoanalytical writings', in J.B. Thompson (ed.) *Paul Ricoeur: Hermeneutics and the Human Sciences*. London: Cambridge University Press.

Rigby, P. (1968) 'Joking relationships, kin categories and clanship among the Gogo'. *Africa* 38, 13s–54.

—— (1975) 'Prophets, diviners, and prophetism: the recent history of Kiganda religion', *Journal of Anthropological Research* 31 (1): 116–48.

Roheim, G. (1934) *The Riddle of the Sphinx or Human Origins*. London: The Hogarth Press.

—— (1945) *The Eternal Ones of the Dream: A Psychoanalytic Interpretation of Australian Myth and Ritual*. New York: International Universities Press.

Rosaldo, M.Z. (1980) *Knowledge and Passion: Ilongot Notions of Self and Social Life*. Cambridge: Cambridge University Press.

Rosaldo, R. (1980) *llongot Headhunting 1883–1974: A study in Society and History*. Stanford: Stanford University Press.

Ruel, M. (1985) 'Growing the girl'. *Cambridge Anthropology* 15: 45–55.

Sahlins, M. (1972) *Stone Age Economics*. Chicago: Aldine.

Sargant, W. (1957) *Battle for the Mind: A Physiology of Conversion and Brainwashing*. London: Heinemann.

Schachter, S. and Singer, J. E. (1962) 'Cognitive, social and physiological determinants of emotional state'. *Psychological Review* 69: 379–99.

Scheff, T.J. (1977) 'The distancing of emotion in ritual'. *Current Anthropology* 18: 483–505.

Schneider, D. (1968) *American Kinship: A Cultural Account*. Englewood Cliffs: Prentice-Hall.

Sharman, A. (1969) 'Joking in Padhola: categorical relationships, choice and social control'. *Man n.s.* 4: 103–17.

Shaver, K.G. (1975) *An Introduction to Attribution Processes*. Cambridge, MA: Winthrop.

Solomon, R.C. (1984) 'Getting angry: the Jamesian theory of emotion in anthropology', in R.A. Shweder and R.A. Levine (eds) *Culture Theory: Essays on Mind, Self and Emotion*. Cambridge: Cambridge University Press.

Southall, A.W. (1960a) 'Homicide and suicide among the Alur', in B. Bohannan (ed.) *African Homicide and Suicide*. Princeton, NJ: Princeton University Press.

—— (1960b) 'On Chastity in Africa'. *Uganda Journal* 24: 207–16.

—— (1970) 'The illusion of tribe'. *Journal of Asian and African Studies* 5: 1–12, 28–50.

Spencer, P. (1965) *The Samburu. A study of Geroniocracy in a Nomadic Tribe.* London: Routledge & Kegan Paul.

—— (1970) 'The function of ritual in the socialization of the Samburu Moran', in P. Mayer (ed.) *Socialization: the Approach from Social Anthropology.* London: Tavistock.

Spiro, M.E. (1982) *Oedipus in the Trobriands.* London and Chicago: University of Chicago Press.

Stanner, W.E.H. (1963) *On Aboriginal Religion.* Oceania Monograph 11, Sydney: University of Sydney Press.

Stephens, W.N. and D'Andrade, R.G. (1962) 'Kin-avoidance', in W.N. Stephens (ed.) *The Oedipus Complex: Cross-cultural evidence.* Glencoe: The Free Press.

Stevens, P. (1978) 'Bachama joking categones: towards new perspectives in the study of joking relationships'. *Journal of Anthropological Research* 34: 47–71.

Sundkler, B. (1948) *Bantu Prophets in South Africa.* London: Lutterworth Press.

Tew, M. (1953) 'A further note on funeral friendships'. *Africa* 21: 122–4.

Thompson, S. (1990) 'Speaking "truth" to power: Divination as a paradigm for facilitating change among the Giriama'. Unpublished PhD thesis, London.

Turner, V.W. (1957) *Schism and Continuity in an African Society.* Manchester: Manchester University Press.

—— (1967) 'Symbols in Ndembu Ritual', in *Forest of Symbols.* Ithaca, NY: Cornell University Press.

—— (1969) 'Symbolisation and patterning in the circumcision rites of two Bantu-speaking societies', in M. Douglas and P. Kaberry (eds) *Man in Africa.* London: Tavistock Press.

—— (1975) *Revelation and Divination in Ndembu Ritual.* Ithaca, NY: Cornell University Press.

Twaddle, M. (1969) 'Tribalism in Eastern Uganda', in P. Gulliver (ed.) *Tradition and Transition in East Africa.* London: Routledge & Kegan Paul.

Vail, L. (1997) 'The invention of tribalism in Southern Africa', in R. Grinkler and C. Steiner (eds) *Perspectives on Africa.* Oxford: Basil Blackwell.

Vansina, J. (1990) *Paths in the Rainforest.* London: James Currey.

Wagner, G. (1940) 'The Political Organisation of the Bantu of Kavirondo', in E.E. Evans-Pritchard and M. Fortes (eds) *African Political Systems.* Oxford: Oxford University Press.

Wangusa, T. (1989) *Upon This Mountain.* London: Heinemann.

Watson, P. (1980) *War on the Mind: Military uses and abuses of psychology.* Harmondsworth: Penguin.

White, L. (1990) *The Comforts of Home: Prostitution in Colonial Nairobi.* Chicago: University of Chicago Press.

—— (1994) 'Blood Brotherhood revisited: Kinship, relationship, and the body in East and Central Africa'. *Africa* 64: 359–72.

Whiting, J.W., Kluckhohn, R. and Anthony, A. (1958) 'The function of male initiation ceremonies at puberty', in E. Maccoby, W. Newcomb and R. Hartley (eds) *Readings in Social Psychology*. New York: Holt, Reinhart and Winston.

Whyte, S.R. (1988) 'Knowledge and Power in Nyole Divination', paper given to the Satterthwaite Colloquium on African Religions.

—— (1990) 'The Widow's Dream: Sex and Death in Western Kenya', in M. Jackson and I. Karp (eds) *Personhood and Agency: The Presentation of Self and Other in African Cultures*. Uppsala: Acta Universitatis Upsaliensis.

Wilson, M. (1957) *Rituals of Kinship among the Nyakyusa*. Oxford: Oxford University Press.

Wolf, J. de. (1977) *Differentiation and Integration in Western Kenya*. The Hague: Mouton.

Young, M. (1971) 'Knowledge and control', in M. Young (ed.) *Knowledge and Control*. London: Collier-Macmillan.

INDEX